THE SIMPLE 30-MINUTE FIBROMYALGIA DIET COOKBOOK

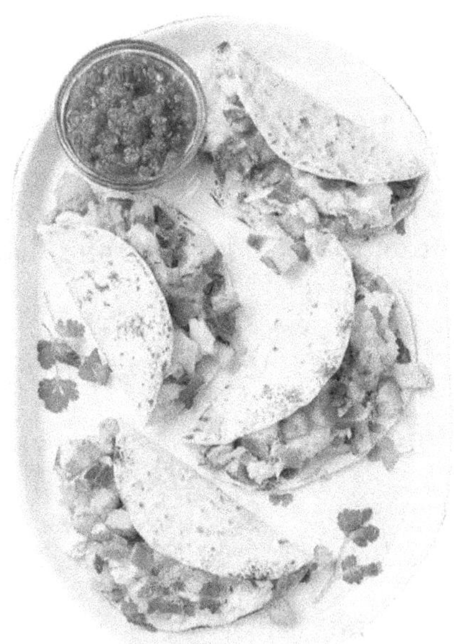

Healthy Delicious Anti-inflammatory Recipes to Cook in Less Than 30 Minutes a Meal

Joan G. Milone

Copyright © 2024 by Joan G. Milone

All rights reserved.

This book is written as a source of information only. The information contained in this book is provided in good faith and is believed to be accurate and reliable as of the date of publication. The author does not assume any responsibility for any errors or omissions that may appear.

To use "The Simple 30-Minute Fibromyalgia Diet Cookbook" effectively:

1. **Read the Introduction**: Understand the diet's principles and how it helps fibromyalgia.

2. **Plan Meals**: Select recipes that fit your taste and schedule.

3. **Shop for Ingredients**: Buy fresh, unprocessed ingredients as listed.

4. **Cook**: Prepare meals according to the cookbook instructions.

5. **Adjust**: Note how foods affect your symptoms and adjust your diet accordingly.

Table of Contents

Introduction 7

Understanding Fibromyalgia: Symptoms, Causes, and Diet's Role 9

The Importance of Nutrition in Managing Fibromyalgia 12

The Psychological Aspect of Nutrition 14

Tips for Quick and Healthy Cooking 14

Chapter 1: Breakfast 17

Anti-Inflammatory Smoothie Bowls 17

Quick Spinach and Feta Scrambled Eggs 19

Overnight Oats with Berries and Chia Seeds 21

Avocado Toast with Poached Eggs 24

Quinoa Porridge with Almonds and Honey 26

Chapter 2: Lunch 29

Turmeric Chicken Salad Wrap 29

Quick Lentil and Vegetable Soup 32

Chickpea and Avocado Salad 34

Quinoa and Black Bean Stuffed Peppers 36

Easy Salmon and Avocado Salad 38

Chapter 3: Dinner   41

Garlic Ginger Shrimp Stir-Fry   41

Lemon Herb Baked Cod   44

Chicken and Broccoli Alfredo (Gluten-Free)   46

Zucchini Noodles with Pesto and Cherry Tomatoes   48

Spicy Tofu and Mushroom Bowl   51

Chapter 4: Snacks and Sides   55

Cucumber and Hummus Bites   55

Sweet Potato and Kale Chips   57

Almond and Flaxseed Energy Balls   60

Quinoa Tabbouleh   62

Baked Zucchini Fries   64

Chapter 5: Seafoods and Fish   67

Pan-Seared Scallops with Lemon Butter Sauce   67

Quick Spicy Salmon Tacos   70

Shrimp Avocado Mango Salad   72

Tilapia with Mango Salsa   74

Garlic Lemon Tuna Patties   76

Chapter 6: Meat and Poultry — 79

Turkey and Spinach Meatballs — 79

Chicken and Quinoa Soup — 81

Balsamic Glazed Steak Rolls — 83

Quick Chicken Parmesan — 86

Spiced Lamb Chops with Yogurt Sauce — 88

Chapter 7: Desserts — 91

Avocado Chocolate Mousse — 91

Coconut Flour Pancakes with Berry Compote — 93

Baked Apples with Cinnamon and Nuts — 96

Quick Mango and Chia Seed Pudding — 98

Honey Roasted Pears with Yogurt — 100

Chapter 8: Soups — 103

Carrot Ginger Soup — 103

Tomato and Basil Soup — 106

Chicken Zoodle Soup — 108

Spicy Pumpkin Soup — 110

Broccoli and Pea Soup with Mint — 112

Chapter 9: Salads 115

Spinach and Strawberry Salad with Walnuts 115

Mediterranean Quinoa Salad 117

Beetroot and Goat Cheese Salad 120

Kale, Avocado, and Quinoa Salad 122

Cucumber Noodle Prawn Salad 124

Chapter 10: Implementing a Fibromyalgia-Friendly Diet 127

7 Days Sample Meal Plan 128

Meal Planning and Preparation Tips 130

Understanding Food Labels and Ingredients to Avoid 132

Staying Hydrated and Other Lifestyle Tips 135

Supplements and Nutrients of Interest for Fibromyalgia 138

Tips for Supplementation 140

Shopping List for a Fibromyalgia-Friendly Pantry 141

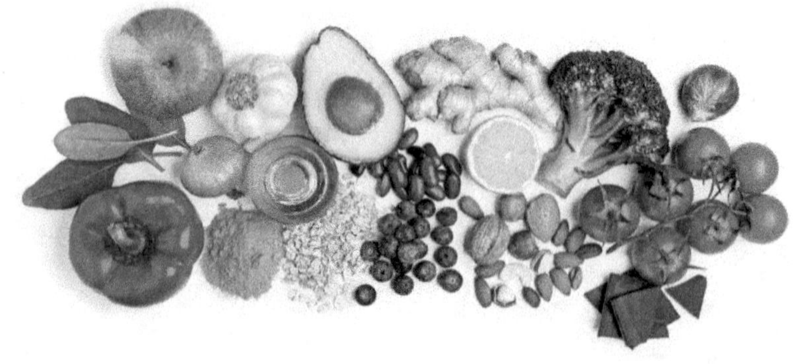

Introduction

Imagine a world in which controlling fibromyalgia does not include negotiating a complex maze of drugs, exhausting therapies, and drastic lifestyle changes. Consider a solution that is so simple and accessible that it fits perfectly into your demanding schedule, taking no more than thirty minutes of your time per stage. Welcome to "The Simple 30-Minute Fibromyalgia Diet Cookbook," your new friend in combating fibromyalgia's chronic symptoms.

As someone who knows the everyday hardships and acute, often devastating pain that fibromyalgia can cause, I've always looked for solutions to ease these symptoms, not just for myself, but for the numerous others who share this path. This book was inspired by a profoundly personal desire to take control of a condition that frequently leaves us feeling powerless. During my journey, I realized that one of the most effective methods to battle fibromyalgia is not in the medicine cabinet, but in the kitchen.

Imagine digging into a selection of dishes that are so tasty and simple to make that you won't believe they're intended to treat fibromyalgia. Each food has been thoughtfully designed, not just for its nutritional content, but also for its ability to be prepared in 30 minutes or less. This is more than simply a cookbook; it is a starting point for a new way of life in which treating your symptoms does not have to take precedence over your life.

Through the pages of "The Simple 30-Minute Fibromyalgia Diet Cookbook," you will embark on a gastronomic journey that does not require you to be a chef or nutritionist. There won't be any scary lists of unusual ingredients here. Instead, you'll find a treasure trove of clean, easy-to-source foods that work in tandem with your body to reduce inflammation, increase energy, and relieve pain.

But this book contains more than simply recipes. It's a narrative of change and optimism. It's about rediscovering the joy of cooking, about meals that nourish the body while also comforting and delighting the spirit. Each page is filled with ideas, tactics, and personal experiences that will teach you not only how to cook, but also how to live a richer, more vibrant life with fibromyalgia.

Join me on this trip. Allow "The Simple 30-Minute Fibromyalgia Diet Cookbook" to change the way you approach your symptoms. We'll look at the power of simple, healthy meals that not only nourish but also heal and inspire. This is more than just a book; it's a guide on the path to wellness, demonstrating that living with fibromyalgia does not have to mean living in pain.

Your journey to a better, happier life begins here. Each dish is more than just cooking; it is a step toward reclaiming your life. Let's turn the page together and find a delightful, uncomplicated way to manage fibromyalgia. Welcome to your fresh beginnings. Hello and thank you for visiting "The Simple 30-Minute Fibromyalgia Diet Cookbook."

Understanding Fibromyalgia: Symptoms, Causes, and Diet's Role

Fibromyalgia is a complicated and sometimes misunderstood disorder marked by widespread chronic pain, exhaustion, sleep difficulties, and other symptoms that differ in intensity and duration from person to person. It's a disorder that's perplexed healthcare specialists for years, with causes thought to be as varied as the symptoms.

Fibromyalgia Symptoms

Fibromyalgia is characterized by chronic, widespread pain that affects numerous sections of the body. This pain is defined as a continuous dull aching that often originates in the muscles and soft tissue. Beyond pain, people with fibromyalgia may experience:

- Profound weariness, even after enough rest.
- Sleep problems include difficulties falling or staying asleep.

- Cognitive impairments, frequently referred to as "fibro fog," impact concentration and memory.
- Mood disorders, such as anxiety and sadness
- Sensitivity to light, sound, and temperature

Causes of Fibromyalgia

Fibromyalgia's specific etiology is unknown, but experts believe it stems from a mix of genetic, environmental, and psychological factors. Some of the possible causes and contributory variables are:

Genetic predisposition: Fibromyalgia often runs in families, suggesting that genetic factors may increase the risk of developing the condition.

Physical or mental trauma: Accidents, surgeries, or major psychological stress can all cause fibromyalgia.

Infections: Some infections tend to worsen or induce fibromyalgia.

Disruptions in pain signals: Abnormalities in how the brain interprets pain signals can cause unpleasant feelings to be amplified.

Diet and Fibromyalgia

While there is no treatment for fibromyalgia, there are ways to manage its symptoms, and nutrition is an important part of that plan. Nutritional therapies can assist with some symptoms by lowering inflammation, improving sleep quality, and increasing energy. Here's how nutrition affects fibromyalgia treatment:

Anti-inflammatory foods: Consuming foods high in omega-3 fatty acids, such as salmon, flaxseeds, and walnuts, can help decrease inflammation and discomfort. Fruits, vegetables, and whole grains are also good anti-inflammatory foods.

Avoiding trigger foods: Certain foods and additives can increase fibromyalgia symptoms in certain people. Processed meals, sugar, coffee, and alcohol are all common contributors. Identifying and removing these triggers can greatly minimize symptoms.

Balanced nutrition: A well-rounded diet provides the body with critical vitamins and minerals, promoting overall health and wellness. Individuals with fibromyalgia require essential nutrients such as vitamin D, magnesium, and B vitamins.

Hydration: Staying hydrated is essential for controlling fibromyalgia. Water helps to remove toxins from the body, lowers inflammation, and boosts energy levels.

Understanding fibromyalgia necessitates comprehending its complexities and the variety of its effects on people. While the reasons for the disorder are unknown, treating its symptoms with a comprehensive strategy that includes dietary changes provides hope to individuals affected. Individuals with fibromyalgia can significantly improve their quality of life by following a balanced, anti-inflammatory diet and recognizing personal dietary triggers.

The Importance of Nutrition in Managing Fibromyalgia

Fibromyalgia, a chronic disorder marked by widespread pain, exhaustion, and a variety of other symptoms, requires a complex approach that includes medicine, physical therapy, and lifestyle changes. Nutrition, for example, plays a key part in efficiently controlling the illness, although is frequently disregarded. The relationship between nutrition and fibromyalgia symptoms is complicated, but recognizing and using this connection may dramatically improve the quality of life for people affected.

Nutritional Effects on Fibromyalgia Symptoms

Nutrition affects fibromyalgia symptoms in a variety of ways. Certain meals might worsen symptoms, while others can help alleviate them. Here's how.

Inflammation: Fibromyalgia is linked to inflammation. Diets rich in anti-inflammatory foods, such as omega-3 fatty acids found in fish and flaxseeds, antioxidants in fruits and vegetables, and polyphenols in green tea, can help reduce inflammation and discomfort.

Fibromyalgia Diet

Gut Health: Emerging evidence indicates a relationship between fibromyalgia and gastrointestinal health. A fiber-rich diet, together with probiotics (found in yogurt and fermented foods) and prebiotics (found in garlic, onions, and bananas), can enhance gut health and perhaps reduce fibromyalgia symptoms.

Fibromyalgia-related tiredness can be severe. A well-balanced diet rich in complex carbs, lean proteins, and healthy fats will help control energy dips and increase overall vitality.

Food Sensitivity: Some fibromyalgia patients report sensitivity to certain foods or additives, which might cause symptoms. Identifying and avoiding triggers, which frequently include gluten, dairy, sugar, and some preservatives, might be critical for symptom management.

Implementing Nutritional Strategies.

Making dietary adjustments might be difficult, but with the appropriate approach, you can establish a nutrition plan that improves fibromyalgia treatment.

Consultation with a Nutritionist: Working with a healthcare practitioner, particularly a dietitian or nutritionist who understands fibromyalgia, can assist you in developing a tailored food plan that meets your individual symptoms and nutritional requirements.

Gradual Changes: It might be overwhelming to completely overhaul your diet overnight. Begin by making tiny, doable adjustments, such as increasing your consumption of fruits and vegetables, eating more whole meals, and progressively removing recognized triggers.

Keeping A Food Diary: Tracking what you eat and how it impacts your symptoms may be really useful. Over time, patterns may form that can guide future dietary changes.

The Psychological Aspect of Nutrition

Beyond the physical effects of eating on fibromyalgia, there is a psychological component. A good diet can boost one's feelings of well-being, control, and optimism. Managing fibromyalgia symptoms with nutrition gives people a sense of control over their health.

The significance of diet in controlling fibromyalgia cannot be emphasized. While not a cure, nutritional choices can considerably reduce symptoms, increase energy, and improve general quality of life. This method, when combined with medical therapy and lifestyle changes, provides a holistic plan for treating fibromyalgia and living a more comfortable, fulfilled life.

Tips for Quick and Healthy Cooking

Quick and healthful cooking is critical for keeping a balanced diet in our hectic lives. Here are some practical methods for preparing nutritious meals efficiently:

Plan Ahead: Take some time each week to plan your meals. This reduces the stress of making last-minute selections and ensures you have the appropriate components on hand.

Keep It Simple: Select recipes that require fewer ingredients and processes. Dishes that may be prepared in a single pot or skillet also save time and effort.

Preparation in Advance: When you have some free time, pre-cut veggies, marinate meats, and measure dry ingredients. On busy days, store them in the refrigerator or freezer to make assembling and cooking easier.

Stock a Healthy Pantry: Keep your pantry, fridge, and freezer stocked with healthy staples like whole grains, canned beans, frozen vegetables, and lean proteins. Having these essentials at hand makes it easier to throw together a nutritious meal.

Use Shortcuts: Don't be afraid to use pre-cut veggies, pre-cooked grains, or canned items like tomatoes and beans (preferably low-sodium varieties). These can drastically save preparation time.

Cook in Batches: When you have the time, prepare dishes in large amounts. Leftovers may be refrigerated or frozen and are ideal for fast future dinners.

Embrace Quick Cooking Methods: Techniques such as stir-frying, steaming, and grilling are not only quick but also maintain nutritious value.

Make Use of Appliances: Slow cookers and pressure cookers may make food preparation easier. These machines cook for you, freeing up your time for other chores.

Dress It Up: Keep a variety of spices, herbs, and condiments on hand to easily add flavor to even the most basic recipes without adding too many calories.

Combine Fresh and Convenience Foods: For a healthy and time-saving meal, combine fresh produce and convenience foods. For a quick and balanced supper, try adding fresh veggies to rotisserie chicken.

Smart Snacking: Make nutritious snacks in advance, such as chopped veggies with hummus, fruit with nut butter, or Greek yogurt with berries, so you can grab and go when you're short on time.

Learn to Love Leftovers: Be creative with leftovers and use them as the foundation for new dinners. For example, use last night's roasted veggies as a substantial omelet or salad topper.

Quick and nutritious cooking is all about making wise decisions and utilizing time-saving tactics to help you achieve your wellness objectives.

Chapter 1: Breakfast

Beginning the day with a nutritious breakfast is crucial for symptom management and sustained energy. This section offers a variety of quick, anti-inflammatory breakfast options designed to meet the dietary needs of fibromyalgia patients. With recipes that are easy to prepare in 30 minutes or less, our focus is on meals rich in nutrients, balanced in proteins, healthy fats, and complex carbohydrates. From antioxidant-packed smoothie bowls to protein-rich egg dishes, these breakfasts are tailored to provide you with the best start to your day, aiming to reduce inflammation, support digestive health, and stabilize blood sugar levels. Dive into these versatile and customizable recipes to nourish your body and support your health journey right from the morning.

Anti-Inflammatory Smoothie Bowls

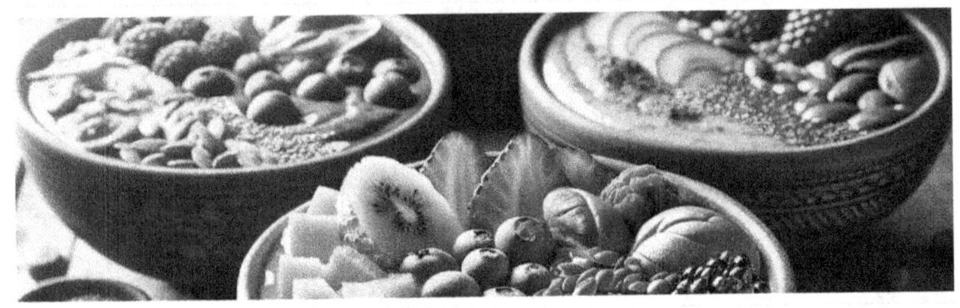

Ingredients:

- 1 cup frozen mixed berries (such as blueberries, strawberries, and raspberries
- 1 small ripe banana
- 1/2 cup baby spinach leaves
- 1 tablespoon chia seeds
- 1 tablespoon flaxseed meal
- 1/2 teaspoon turmeric powder
- 1/4 teaspoon ground ginger
- 1 cup unsweetened almond milk (or any plant-based milk of choice)
- Optional toppings: sliced almonds, fresh berries, unsweetened coconut flakes, granola

Preparation:

1. In a blender, combine the frozen berries, banana, baby spinach, chia seeds, flaxseed meal, turmeric powder, and ground ginger.
2. Pour in the almond milk and blend on high until smooth and creamy.
3. Pour the smoothie into bowls and garnish with your choice of toppings such as sliced almonds, fresh berries, coconut flakes, and granola for added texture and nutrients.

Nutritional Value:

- Calories: Approximately 300 kcal per serving (without toppings)
- Protein: 6g
- Fat: 7g (Healthy fats from chia seeds, flaxseed, and almond milk)
- Carbohydrates: 50g
- Fiber: 12g
- Sugars: 20g (Natural sugars from fruits)
- Rich in antioxidants, omega-3 fatty acids, and vitamins A, C, and E from the fruits and seeds, which are beneficial for reducing inflammation.

Cooking Time:

- Preparation time: 5 minutes
- Total time: 5 minutes

Rating: ★★★★★

This Anti-Inflammatory Smoothie Bowl is not just a delight to the taste buds but also a powerful tool in combating inflammation, thanks to its high antioxidant content and nutrient-dense ingredients. It's a perfect, quick, and easy breakfast option for anyone looking to support their health, particularly for those managing fibromyalgia.

Quick Spinach and Feta Scrambled Eggs

Ingredients:

- 4 large eggs

- 1/4 cup milk (any variety to suit dietary needs)
- 1/2 cup fresh spinach, roughly chopped
- 1/4 cup feta cheese, crumbled
- Salt and pepper to taste
- 1 tablespoon olive oil or butter

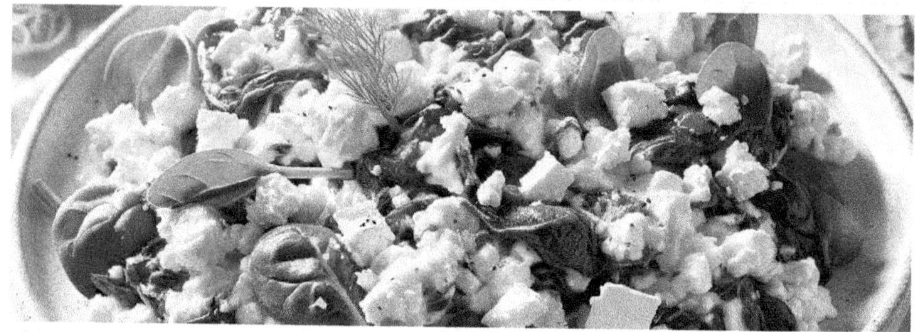

Preparation:

1. In a bowl, whisk together the eggs, milk, salt, and pepper until well combined.
2. Heat olive oil or butter in a non-stick skillet over medium heat.
3. Add the chopped spinach to the skillet and sauté for 1-2 minutes until slightly wilted.
4. Pour the egg mixture over the spinach. Allow it to sit for a few seconds until it begins to set around the edges.
5. Gently stir the eggs and spinach, scraping the bottom of the skillet, until the eggs are softly set.
6. Sprinkle the crumbled feta cheese over the eggs, and fold gently to combine. Cook for an additional minute, or until the cheese is slightly melted and the eggs are cooked to your liking.

7. Serve immediately.

Nutritional Value (per serving):

- Calories: Approximately 250 kcal
- Protein: 18g
- Fat: 18g (healthy fats from olive oil and feta cheese)
- Carbohydrates: 3g
- Fiber: 0.5g
- High in vitamins A and C from spinach, calcium from feta cheese, and omega-3 fatty acids from eggs.

Cooking Time:

- Preparation time: 5 minutes
- Cook time: 5 minutes
- Total time: 10 minutes

Rating: ★★★★★

This Quick Spinach and Feta Scrambled Eggs recipe is a healthy, flavorful, and easy-to-make breakfast option. Packed with protein, healthy fats, and essential vitamins, it's perfect for anyone looking to start their day with a nutritious meal. The combination of fresh spinach and tangy feta adds a delicious Mediterranean twist to your morning eggs.

Overnight Oats with Berries and Chia Seeds

Ingredients:

- 1/2 cup rolled oats

- 3/4 cup almond milk (or any plant-based milk of your choice)
- 1 tablespoon chia seeds
- 1/2 teaspoon vanilla extract
- 1 tablespoon maple syrup or honey (adjust to taste)
- 1/2 cup mixed berries (fresh or frozen)
- Optional toppings: additional berries, sliced almonds, hemp seeds, a dollop of yogurt

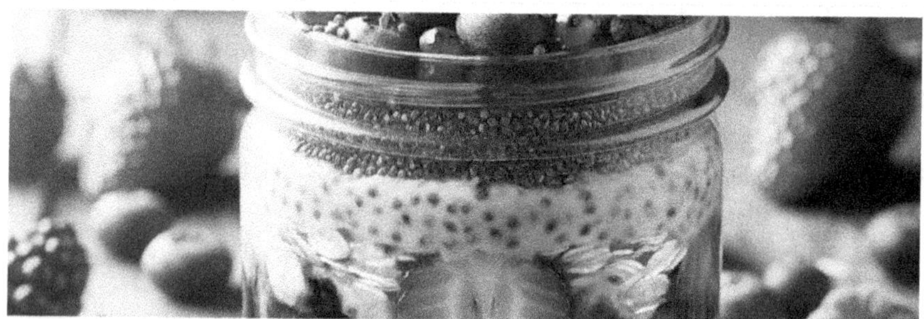

Preparation:

1. In a mason jar or airtight container, combine the rolled oats, almond milk, chia seeds, vanilla extract, and maple syrup or honey. Stir well to mix all the ingredients.
2. Gently fold in the mixed berries.
3. Seal the container and refrigerate overnight, or for at least 6 hours, allowing the oats and chia seeds to absorb the liquid and soften.

4. Before serving, stir the oats well. If the mixture is too thick, you can add a little more almond milk to reach your desired consistency.

5. Garnish with additional berries, sliced almonds, hemp seeds, or a dollop of yogurt, if desired.

Nutritional Value (per serving):

- Calories: Approximately 300-350 kcal (varies with toppings)
- Protein: 8g
- Fat: 7g (healthy fats from chia seeds)
- Carbohydrates: 55g
- Fiber: 10g
- Sugars: 15g (natural sugars from berries and added sweetener)
- Rich in omega-3 fatty acids from chia seeds, antioxidants from berries, and fiber from oats, making it a heart-healthy and digestion-friendly breakfast option.

Cooking Time:

- Preparation time: 5 minutes (plus overnight soaking)
- Total time: 5 minutes active, 6+ hours passive

Rating: ★★★★★

Overnight Oats with Berries and Chia Seeds is a perfect breakfast for those on the go. It's not only delicious and satisfying but also packed with nutrients that support overall health, including fiber for digestion, omega-3 fatty acids for heart health, and antioxidants for immune support. This make-ahead meal is a convenient and healthy option for busy mornings or when you need a quick and nourishing start to your day.

Avocado Toast with Poached Eggs

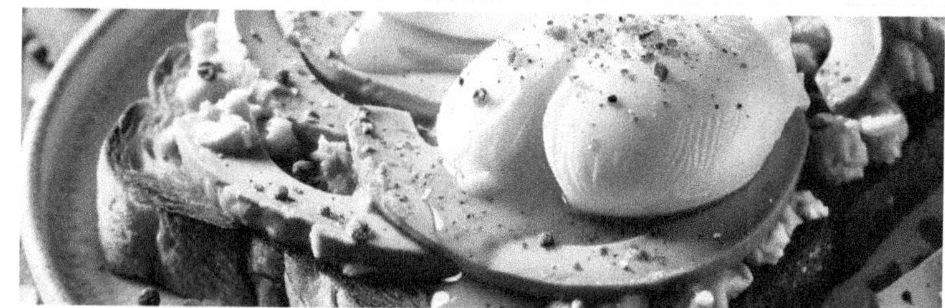

Ingredients:

- 2 slices of whole grain or sourdough bread
- 1 ripe avocado
- 2 eggs
- Salt and pepper to taste
- 1 tablespoon white vinegar (for poaching eggs)
- Optional garnishes: chili flakes, fresh herbs (such as cilantro or parsley), a squeeze of lemon juice

Preparation:

1. Toast the bread slices to your preferred level of crispiness.

2. Cut the avocado in half, remove the pit, and scoop the flesh into a bowl. Mash the avocado with a fork and season with salt and pepper. Spread the mashed avocado evenly onto the toasted bread slices.

3. To poach the eggs, bring a pot of water to a gentle simmer and add the white vinegar. Crack each egg into a small bowl or cup. Gently slide the eggs into the simmering water one at a time. Cook for about 3-4 minutes for soft poached eggs or longer for firmer yolks.

4. Use a slotted spoon to remove the eggs from the water and drain them on a kitchen towel.

5. Place a poached egg on top of each avocado toast. Season with salt and pepper, and add any optional garnishes like chili flakes, fresh herbs, or a squeeze of lemon juice.

Nutritional Value (per serving):

- Calories: Approximately 300-350 kcal
- Protein: 12g
- Fat: 20g (healthy fats from avocado)
- Carbohydrates: 27g
- Fiber: 9g
- Rich in vitamins E and C, potassium from the avocado, and omega-3 fatty acids from the eggs.

Cooking Time:

- Preparation time: 10 minutes
- Cook time: 5 minutes
- Total time: 15 minutes

Rating: ★★★★★

Avocado Toast with Poached Eggs combines the creamy texture of ripe avocado with the richness of a perfectly poached egg, all atop a crispy slice of toast. This dish is not only visually appealing but also packed with nutrients, offering a balanced blend of healthy fats, proteins, and fibers. It's a simple yet sophisticated breakfast option that's perfect for starting your day with energy and satisfaction. The addition of optional garnishes can elevate the flavor, making this dish versatile to suit various taste preferences.

Quinoa Porridge with Almonds and Honey

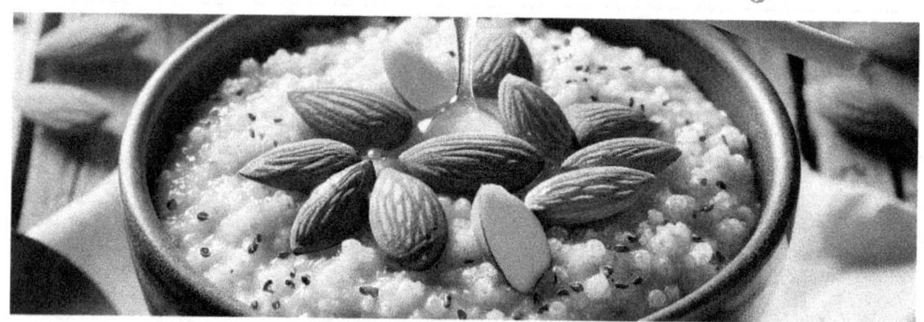

Ingredients:

- 1 cup quinoa, rinsed and drained
- 2 cups almond milk (or any milk of your choice)
- 1/2 teaspoon cinnamon
- Pinch of salt
- 2 tablespoons honey (or to taste)

- 1/4 cup almonds, sliced or chopped
- Optional toppings: fresh berries, sliced banana, chia seeds

Preparation:

1. In a medium saucepan, combine the rinsed quinoa, almond milk, cinnamon, and a pinch of salt. Stir to mix.
2. Bring the mixture to a boil over medium heat, then reduce the heat to low, cover, and simmer for 15-20 minutes, or until most of the liquid is absorbed and the quinoa is tender.
3. Remove from heat and let it stand covered for 5 minutes; the quinoa will absorb any remaining liquid.
4. Stir in the honey, adjusting the amount to your liking for sweetness.
5. Serve the porridge in bowls, topped with sliced almonds and any other optional toppings like fresh berries or sliced banana.

Nutritional Value (per serving):

- Calories: Approximately 250-300 kcal (without additional toppings)
- Protein: 8g
- Fat: 7g (healthy fats from almonds)
- Carbohydrates: 40g
- Fiber: 5g
- Rich in minerals such as magnesium and iron from quinoa, vitamin E from

almonds, and antioxidants from honey.

Cooking Time:

- Preparation time: 5 minutes
- Cook time: 20 minutes
- Total time: 25 minutes

Rating: ★★★★★

Quinoa Porridge with Almonds and Honey is a warm, comforting breakfast that's perfect for starting your day with a nutritious and satisfying meal. This dish not only offers a delicious taste and creamy texture but also provides a wealth of health benefits. Quinoa, a complete protein containing all nine essential amino acids, pairs beautifully with the crunch of almonds and the natural sweetness of honey. This porridge is a fantastic alternative to traditional oatmeal, bringing variety to your morning routine while keeping you energized and full throughout the morning.

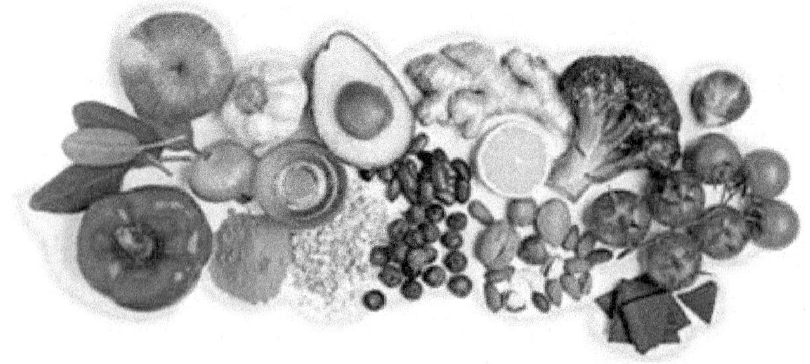

Chapter 2: Lunch

Lunch is your chance to recharge with a meal that's both satisfying and supportive of your health, especially for those treating fibromyalgia. Our lunch recipes are quick, nutritious, and designed to fit into your busy day while helping to ease inflammation and boost your energy. From fresh salads and soups to wraps and bowls, each dish is packed with flavor and essential nutrients. These meals are not just about filling up but nourishing your body to support your health and well-being, whether you're at home or on the go.

Turmeric Chicken Salad Wrap

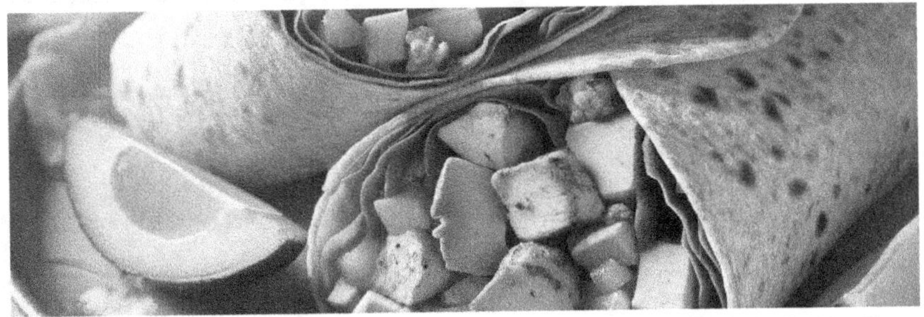

Ingredients:

- 2 boneless, skinless chicken breasts
- 1 teaspoon turmeric powder
- 1/2 teaspoon garlic powder
- Salt and pepper to taste
- 1 tablespoon olive oil
- 2 cups mixed salad greens (such as spinach, arugula, and romaine)
- 1/2 cup grated carrots
- 1/4 cup sliced cucumber
- 1/4 cup cherry tomatoes, halved
- 1/4 cup red onion, thinly sliced
- 2 tablespoons Greek yogurt or mayonnaise
- 1 teaspoon honey
- 1 tablespoon lemon juice
- 4 whole grain or gluten-free tortillas

Preparation:

1. Season the chicken breasts with turmeric, garlic powder, salt, and pepper. Heat olive oil in a skillet over medium heat and cook the chicken for about 5-7 minutes on each side, or until fully cooked and golden. Let it cool, then slice into strips.
2. In a large bowl, combine the mixed salad greens, grated carrots, sliced cucumber, cherry tomatoes, and red onion.
3. In a small bowl, whisk together Greek yogurt (or mayonnaise), honey, and lemon juice to make the dressing. Adjust the seasoning with salt and pepper.
4. Add the dressing to the salad mixture and toss until everything is well coated.

5. Place an equal amount of the salad mixture on each tortilla, top with sliced chicken, and roll up tightly to form a wrap.

Nutritional Value (per wrap):

- Calories: Approximately 300 kcal
- Protein: 25g
- Fat: 9g (healthy fats from olive oil and Greek yogurt)
- Carbohydrates: 27g
- Fiber: 4g
- Turmeric adds anti-inflammatory properties, while the chicken provides lean protein, and the vegetables offer vitamins, minerals, and fiber.

Cooking Time:

- Preparation time: 15 minutes
- Cook time: 15 minutes
- Total time: 30 minutes

Rating: ★★★★★

This Turmeric Chicken Salad Wrap is a flavorful, nutritious meal perfect for a quick lunch. It combines the healing properties of turmeric with the crunch of fresh vegetables and the lean protein from chicken, all wrapped in a convenient and tasty package. Ideal for those seeking a meal that supports health while satisfying hunger, this wrap is a great addition to a fibromyalgia-friendly diet.

Quick Lentil and Vegetable Soup

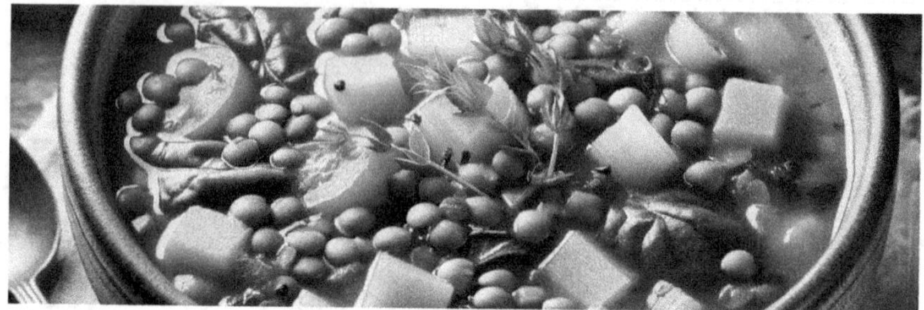

Ingredients:

- 1 tablespoon olive oil
- 1 medium onion, diced
- 2 cloves garlic, minced
- 1 large carrot, diced
- 1 stalk celery, diced
- 1 1/2 cups red lentils, rinsed (red lentils cook faster)
- 1 can (14.5 oz) diced tomatoes, undrained
- 4 cups vegetable broth
- 1 teaspoon ground cumin
- 1/2 teaspoon ground turmeric
- Salt and pepper, to taste
- 2 cups baby spinach, roughly chopped
- 1 tablespoon lemon juice

Preparation:

1. In a large pot, heat olive oil over medium heat. Add onion and garlic, sauté until onion is translucent, about 2-3 minutes.
2. Add carrot and celery; cook until they start to soften, about 5 minutes.

3. Stir in red lentils, diced tomatoes with their juice, vegetable broth, cumin, and turmeric. Season with salt and pepper.

4. Increase heat to high and bring to a boil. Once boiling, reduce heat to a simmer and cover, cooking until lentils are tender, about 15 minutes.

5. Add spinach and cook until wilted, about 2 minutes. Stir in lemon juice and adjust seasoning if necessary.

6. Serve hot.

Nutritional Value (per serving):

- Calories: -220 kcal
- Protein: 14g
- Fat: 3g (healthy fats from olive oil)
- Carbohydrates: 36g
- Fiber: 17g
- This soup is rich in plant-based protein, fiber, vitamins (A, C, K from spinach), and minerals (iron from lentils), with the added anti-inflammatory benefits of turmeric.

Cooking Time:

- Prep Time: 5 minutes
- Cook Time: 20 minutes
- Total Time: 25 minutes

Rating: ★★★★★

This Quick Lentil and Vegetable Soup is an ideal recipe for a nutritious, comforting meal on a tight schedule. Utilizing red lentils reduces cooking time, making it possible to enjoy a wholesome, flavorful soup in under 30 minutes. Perfect for a fibromyalgia-friendly diet or anyone looking for a healthy, quick-to-prepare lunch or dinner option.

Chickpea and Avocado Salad

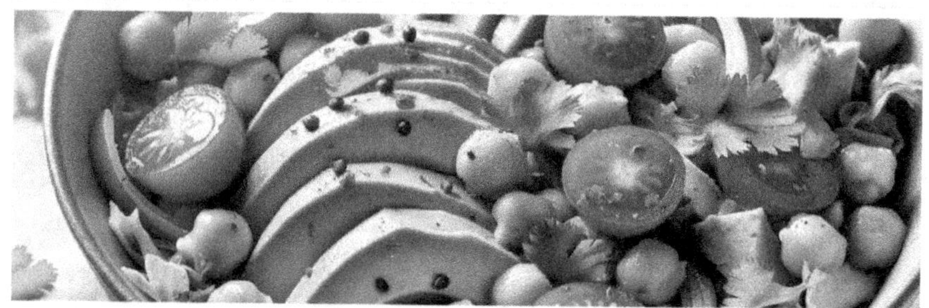

Ingredients:

- 1 can (15 oz) chickpeas, drained and rinsed
- 1 ripe avocado, diced
- 1/2 red onion, finely chopped
- 1/2 cup cherry tomatoes, halved
- 1/4 cup fresh cilantro, chopped (optional)
- 2 tablespoons olive oil
- 1 tablespoon lemon juice
- Salt and pepper to taste
- Optional: 1 cucumber, diced, and 1 bell pepper, diced for extra crunch and nutrition

Preparation:

1. In a large bowl, combine the drained and rinsed chickpeas, diced avocado, chopped red onion, halved cherry tomatoes, and chopped cilantro (if using).
2. In a small bowl, whisk together the olive oil and lemon juice until well combined. Season with salt and pepper to taste.
3. Pour the dressing over the chickpea and avocado mixture. Gently toss to ensure all ingredients are evenly coated with the dressing.
4. Taste and adjust the seasoning if necessary, adding more salt, pepper, or lemon juice as desired.
5. Serve immediately, or let the salad chill in the refrigerator for about 30 minutes to allow the flavors to meld together.

Nutritional Value (per serving):

- Calories: Approximately 250 kcal
- Protein: 7g
- Fat: 14g (healthy fats from avocado and olive oil)
- Carbohydrates: 27g
- Fiber: 9g
- Rich in vitamins C and E, potassium from the avocado, and fiber from the chickpeas. The olive oil adds heart-healthy monounsaturated fats.

Cooking Time:

- Preparation time: 10 minutes
- Total time: 10 minutes

Rating: ★★★★★

This Chickpea and Avocado Salad is a quick, nutritious, and filling dish that's perfect for a healthy lunch. Packed with plant-based protein, fiber, and healthy fats, it's an excellent choice for anyone looking for a meal that supports overall health.

Quinoa and Black Bean Stuffed Peppers

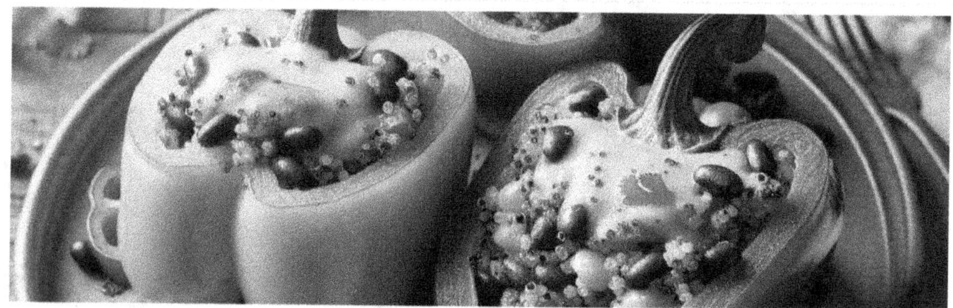

Ingredients:

- 4 large bell peppers, halved and seeds removed
- 1 cup cooked quinoa (use pre-cooked or microwaveable quinoa to save time)
- 1 can (15 oz) black beans, drained and rinsed
- 1 cup corn kernels (use canned or thawed if frozen for convenience)
- 1/2 cup tomato sauce
- 1 teaspoon cumin
- 1/2 teaspoon garlic powder
- 1/2 teaspoon chili powder
- Salt and pepper to taste

- 1/2 cup shredded cheese (optional, can be omitted for a vegan option)
- Fresh cilantro, chopped, for garnish (optional)
- Lime wedges, for serving (optional)

Preparation:

1. Preheat your oven to 375°F (190°C). Arrange the bell pepper halves in a microwave-safe dish, cut-side up. Add a splash of water to the dish, cover with plastic wrap, and microwave on high for 5-7 minutes, or until the peppers are just tender. This step pre-cooks the peppers to save oven time.
2. While the peppers are microwaving, mix the cooked quinoa, black beans, corn, tomato sauce, cumin, garlic powder, chili powder, salt, and pepper in a bowl.
3. Carefully remove the peppers from the microwave, discard any water, and spoon the quinoa mixture into each pepper half.
4. (Optional) Sprinkle with shredded cheese. Place the stuffed peppers in the oven directly on the rack or on a baking sheet for about 10 minutes, or until heated through and the cheese is melted.
5. Garnish with cilantro and serve with lime wedges on the side if desired.

Nutritional Value (approximate per serving):

- Calories: 250 kcal
- Protein: 10g

- Fat: 3g (without cheese)
- Carbohydrates: 45g
- Fiber: 10g

Cooking Time:

- Preparation time: 10 minutes
- Cook time: 15-17 minutes
- Total time: 25-27 minutes

Rating: ★★★★★

This Quick Quinoa and Black Bean Stuffed Peppers recipe is designed to fit into a busy schedule, offering a nutritious and delicious meal in under 30 minutes. By pre-cooking the peppers in the microwave and using pre-cooked quinoa, you save significant preparation and cooking time. This meal remains a wholesome, flavorful option perfect for a quick lunch or dinner.

Easy Salmon and Avocado Salad

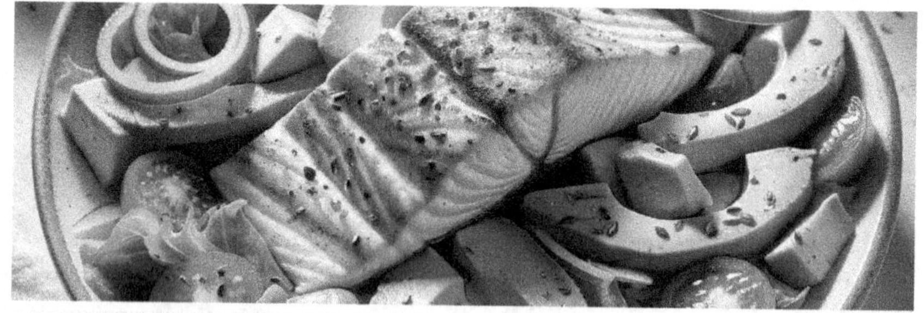

Ingredients:

- 2 salmon fillets (about 4-6 oz each)
- Salt and pepper to taste
- 1 tablespoon olive oil

- 2 ripe avocados, diced
- 1/2 red onion, thinly sliced
- 1/2 cup cherry tomatoes, halved
- 2 cups mixed greens (e.g., arugula, spinach, and baby kale)

For the dressing:

- 2 tablespoons olive oil
- 1 tablespoon lemon juice
- 1 teaspoon Dijon mustard
- Salt and pepper to taste

Preparation:

1. Season the salmon fillets with salt and pepper. Heat 1 tablespoon of olive oil in a pan over medium-high heat. Cook the salmon for 3-4 minutes on each side, or until cooked through and easily flaked with a fork. Remove from the heat and let it cool slightly, then flake into large pieces.

2. In a large bowl, combine the diced avocados, sliced red onion, cherry tomatoes, and mixed greens.

3. Prepare the dressing by whisking together 2 tablespoons of olive oil, lemon juice, Dijon mustard, salt, and pepper in a small bowl.

4. Add the flaked salmon to the salad mixture. Drizzle the dressing over the salad and gently toss to combine, ensuring everything is evenly coated.

5. Serve immediately, optionally garnished with additional lemon wedges or fresh herbs.

Nutritional Value (per serving):

- Calories: Approximately 400-450 kcal
- Protein: 24g
- Fat: 32g (healthy fats from salmon and avocado)
- Carbohydrates: 12g
- Fiber: 7g
- This salad is rich in omega-3 fatty acids, vitamins A and C, potassium, and antioxidants.

Cooking Time:

- Preparation time: 10 minutes
- Cook time: 8 minutes
- Total time: 18 minutes

Rating: ★★★★★

This Easy Salmon and Avocado Salad is a perfect combination of flavors and textures, offering a hearty yet refreshing meal that's ideal for a quick lunch or a light dinner. With the omega-3-rich salmon and the creamy, nutrient-dense avocado, it's not only delicious but also incredibly beneficial for your health, supporting heart health, reducing inflammation, and providing a substantial amount of dietary fiber.

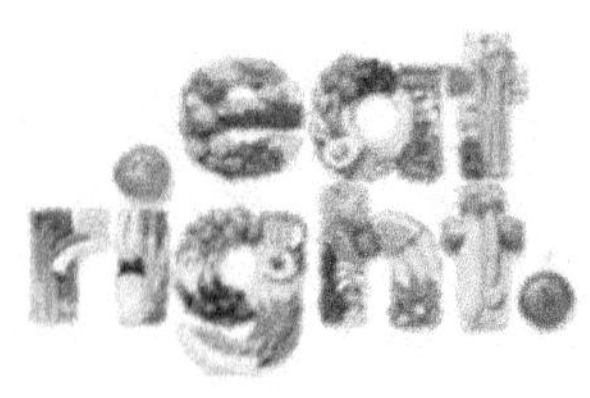

Chapter 3: Dinner

As the day winds down, dinner becomes a crucial meal to nourish your body and comfort your soul, especially for those managing fibromyalgia. This chapter offers a collection of quick, wholesome dinner recipes designed to be prepared in 30 minutes or less. Each meal is crafted to deliver maximum flavor and nutritional benefits, helping to ease inflammation and support your overall well-being. Enjoy ending your day with these simple yet delightful meals that cater to your health and save on your time.

Garlic Ginger Shrimp Stir-Fry

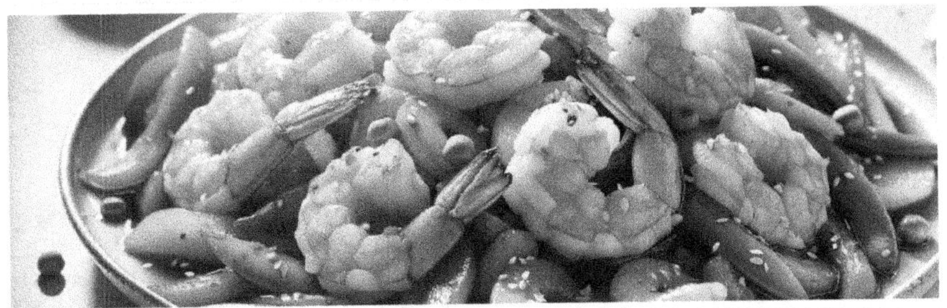

Ingredients:

- 1 pound (450g) shrimp, peeled and deveined

- 2 tablespoons olive oil

- 2 cloves garlic, minced

- 1 tablespoon fresh ginger, minced
- 1 bell pepper, sliced
- 1 cup snap peas
- 1 carrot, julienned
- 2 tablespoons soy sauce (or tamari for gluten-free option)
- 1 tablespoon honey (or maple syrup)
- 1 teaspoon sesame oil
- Salt and pepper to taste
- Optional: sesame seeds and sliced green onions for garnish

Preparation:

1. Heat olive oil in a large skillet or wok over medium-high heat. Add the garlic and ginger, sautéing for about 30 seconds until fragrant.
2. Add the shrimp to the skillet. Cook for 2-3 minutes, or until the shrimp start to turn pink. Remove the shrimp from the skillet and set aside.
3. In the same skillet, add the bell pepper, snap peas, and carrot. Stir-fry for about 5 minutes, or until the vegetables are just tender.
4. In a small bowl, whisk together the soy sauce, honey, and sesame oil. Add this sauce to the skillet with the vegetables, then return the shrimp to the skillet. Stir well to combine and heat through for another 2 minutes. Season with salt and pepper to taste.
5. Garnish with sesame seeds and sliced green onions if desired.

Nutritional Value (per serving):

- Calories: Approximately 220 kcal
- Protein: 24g
- Fat: 8g (healthy fats from olive oil and sesame oil)
- Carbohydrates: 12g
- Fiber: 2g

- This dish is rich in protein, low in carbohydrates, and offers a good source of vitamins and minerals from the vegetables. The ginger and garlic provide anti-inflammatory benefits.

Cooking Time:

- Preparation time: 10 minutes
- Cook time: 10 minutes
- Total time: 20 minutes

Rating: ★★★★★

This Garlic Ginger Shrimp Stir-Fry is a vibrant, flavor-packed dish that comes together in just 20 minutes, making it a perfect dinner option for those busy evenings. It balances the rich flavors of garlic and ginger with the freshness of vegetables and the succulence of shrimp, offering a nutritious meal that supports a healthy lifestyle. Easy to prepare and delightful to eat, this stir-fry is sure to become a staple in your culinary repertoire.

Lemon Herb Baked Cod

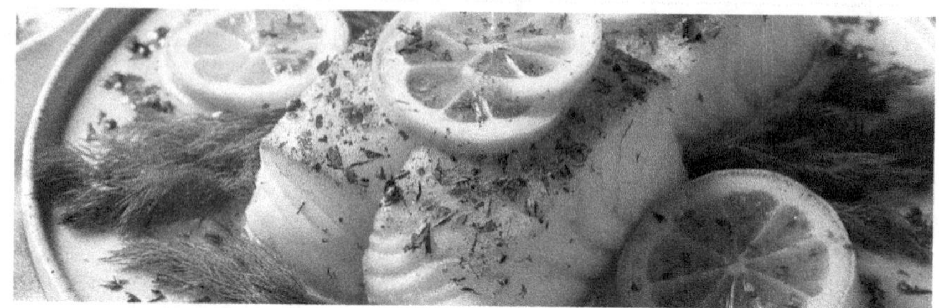

Ingredients:

- 4 cod fillets (about 6 ounces each)
- 2 tablespoons olive oil
- 1 lemon, juiced and zested
- 2 cloves garlic, minced
- 1 tablespoon fresh parsley, finely chopped
- 1 tablespoon fresh dill, finely chopped (or 1 teaspoon dried dill)
- Salt and pepper to taste
- Additional lemon slices for garnish

Preparation:

1. Preheat the oven to 400°F (200°C). Line a baking sheet with parchment paper.

2. In a small bowl, mix together olive oil, lemon juice and zest, minced garlic, chopped parsley, and dill. Season with salt and pepper to taste.

3. Place the cod fillets on the prepared baking sheet. Brush each fillet evenly with the lemon herb mixture.

4. Bake in the preheated oven for 12-15 minutes, or until the fish flakes easily with a fork.

5. Garnish with lemon slices and additional fresh herbs if desired before serving.

Nutritional Value (per serving):

- Calories: Approximately 200 kcal
- Protein: 23g
- Fat: 10g (healthy fats from olive oil)
- Carbohydrates: 2g
- Fiber: 0g
- This dish is an excellent source of high-quality protein and omega-3 fatty acids, beneficial for heart health. The lemon and herbs add a flavorful, antioxidant-rich touch without adding extra calories.

Cooking Time:

- Preparation time: 5 minutes
- Cook time: 15 minutes
- Total time: 20 minutes

Rating: ★★★★★

Lemon Herb Baked Cod is a light, refreshing dish that's perfect for a quick and healthy dinner. The combination of lemon and herbs brings out the delicate flavors of the cod, making it a satisfying meal that's as nutritious as it is delicious. With minimal preparation time and a short cooking duration, this dish is an ideal choice for anyone looking to enjoy a wholesome meal without spending too much time in the kitchen.

Chicken and Broccoli Alfredo (Gluten-Free)

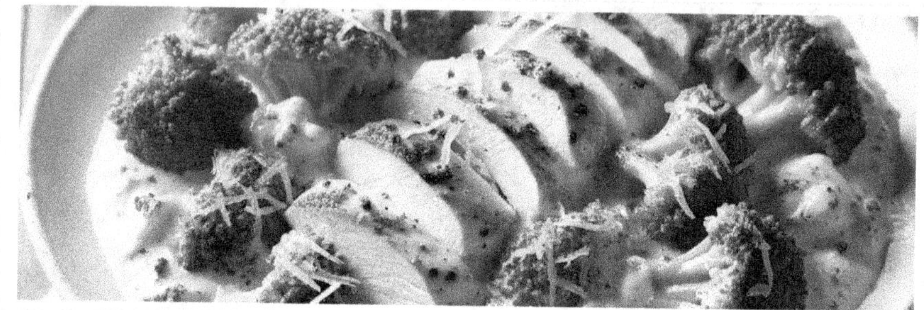

Ingredients:

- 2 large boneless, skinless chicken breasts, cut into bite-sized pieces
- Salt and pepper to taste
- 1 tablespoon olive oil
- 2 cups broccoli florets
- 1 cup heavy cream
- 1/2 cup grated Parmesan cheese, plus more for serving
- 2 cloves garlic, minced
- 8 oz gluten-free fettuccine or any gluten-free pasta of choice
- Optional: red pepper flakes for added heat

Preparation:

1. Cook the gluten-free pasta according to package instructions until al dente. Drain and set aside, reserving 1 cup of pasta water.

2. While the pasta cooks, season the chicken pieces with salt and pepper. Heat olive oil in a large skillet over medium heat. Add the chicken and cook until golden brown and cooked through, about 5-7 minutes. Remove chicken from the skillet and set aside.

3. In the same skillet, add the broccoli florets and a splash of water. Cover and cook until the broccoli is bright green and tender, about 3-4 minutes. Remove the broccoli and set aside with the chicken.

4. In the same skillet, add the minced garlic and sauté for 1 minute until fragrant. Pour in the heavy cream and bring to a simmer. Lower the heat and stir in the grated Parmesan cheese until melted and smooth. If the sauce is too thick, add a bit of the reserved pasta water until you reach the desired consistency.

5. Add the cooked pasta, chicken, and broccoli back into the skillet with the Alfredo sauce. Toss everything together until the pasta is well coated in the sauce. Season with salt, pepper, and red pepper flakes (if using) to taste.

6. Serve hot, garnished with extra Parmesan cheese on top.

Nutritional Value (per serving):

- Calories: Approximately 600 kcal
- Protein: 35g
- Fat: 35g

- Carbohydrates: 45g (varies depending on the type of gluten-free pasta used)
- Fiber: 3g
- This dish offers a good balance of protein from the chicken, vitamins, and minerals from the broccoli, and healthy fats from the cream and Parmesan cheese.

Cooking Time:

- Preparation time: 10 minutes
- Cook time: 20 minutes
- Total time: 30 minutes

Rating: ★★★★★

This Chicken and Broccoli Alfredo is a comforting, creamy, and satisfying dish that's perfect for those following a gluten-free diet. It combines the classic flavors of Alfredo sauce with the nutritional benefits of chicken and broccoli, all made within 30 minutes for a quick and easy dinner option

Zucchini Noodles with Pesto and Cherry Tomatoes

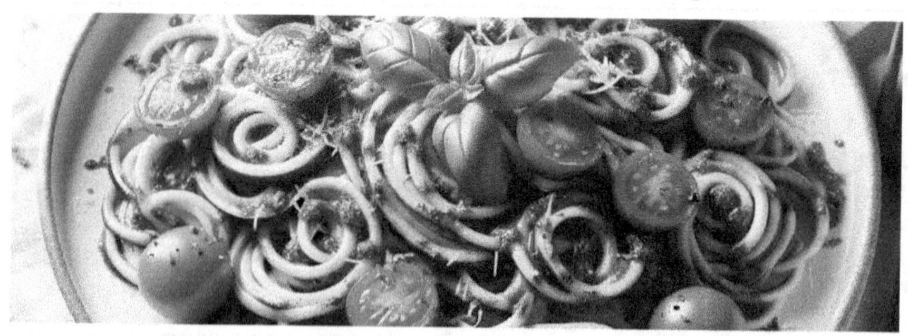

Ingredients:

- 4 medium zucchinis, spiralized into noodles
- 1 cup cherry tomatoes, halved
- 1/2 cup prepared pesto (choose a gluten-free variety if necessary)
- 2 tablespoons olive oil
- Salt and pepper to taste
- Optional garnishes: grated Parmesan cheese, fresh basil leaves, pine nuts

Preparation:

1. Heat 1 tablespoon of olive oil in a large skillet over medium heat. Add the spiralized zucchini noodles (zoodles) and gently sauté for 2-3 minutes, just until tender. Be careful not to overcook to avoid them becoming too soft. Season with salt and pepper to taste.
2. Remove the skillet from the heat. Stir in the pesto until the zoodles are evenly coated.
3. In the same skillet (or another if you prefer), add the remaining tablespoon of olive oil and sauté the cherry tomatoes for about 1-2 minutes, just until they start to soften and release their juices.
4. Toss the sautéed cherry tomatoes with the pesto-coated zoodles. Adjust seasoning if needed.
5. Serve warm, garnished with grated Parmesan cheese, fresh basil leaves, and pine nuts if desired.

Nutritional Value (per serving):

- Calories: Approximately 250 kcal
- Protein: 6g
- Fat: 20g (healthy fats from olive oil and pesto)
- Carbohydrates: 10g
- Fiber: 3g
- This dish is low in carbohydrates and calories, making it a great option for those on a low-carb or ketogenic diet. The zucchini provides vitamins C and A, while the pesto adds a flavorful boost of antioxidants and healthy fats.

Cooking Time:

- Preparation time: 10 minutes
- Cook time: 5 minutes
- Total time: 15 minutes

Rating: ★★★★★

Zucchini Noodles with Pesto and Cherry Tomatoes is a vibrant, fresh, and easy-to-prepare dish perfect for a quick and healthy dinner. This recipe offers a delightful way to enjoy the flavors of summer with minimal cooking time, making it an ideal choice for those seeking a nutritious meal without spending too much time in the kitchen. Light yet satisfying, it's a wonderful alternative to traditional pasta, especially for those looking to reduce their carbohydrate intake.

Spicy Tofu and Mushroom Bowl

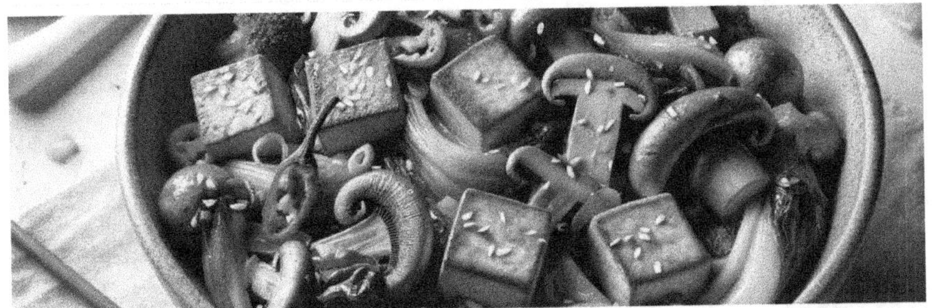

Ingredients:

- 14 oz (400g) firm tofu, pressed and cubed
- 2 cups mushrooms, sliced (e.g., shiitake, cremini, or button)
- 1 tablespoon olive oil
- 2 tablespoons soy sauce (or tamari for a gluten-free option)
- 1 tablespoon chili sauce or sriracha (adjust according to spice preference)
- 1 teaspoon garlic powder
- 1 teaspoon ginger powder
- 2 cups cooked brown rice or quinoa
- 1 cup spinach or kale, roughly chopped
- Optional garnishes: sliced green onions, sesame seeds, fresh cilantro

Preparation:

1. Heat the olive oil in a large skillet over medium-high heat. Add the tofu cubes and sauté until they are golden brown on all sides, about 5-7 minutes.

2. Add the sliced mushrooms to the skillet with the tofu. Cook until the mushrooms are soft and browned, about 5 minutes.

3. In a small bowl, mix together the soy sauce, chili sauce, garlic powder, and ginger powder. Pour this mixture over the tofu and mushrooms in the skillet. Stir well to coat all the pieces evenly. Cook for an additional 2-3 minutes, allowing the flavors to meld together.

4. In the meantime, prepare your bowls by dividing the cooked brown rice or quinoa and chopped spinach or kale between them.

5. Spoon the spicy tofu and mushroom mixture over the rice or quinoa. Garnish with sliced green onions, sesame seeds, and fresh cilantro if desired.

Nutritional Value (per serving):

- Calories: Approximately 350 kcal
- Protein: 18g
- Fat: 12g (healthy fats from olive oil and tofu)
- Carbohydrates: 45g (if served with brown rice)
- Fiber: 6g
- This dish is high in protein, fiber, and essential nutrients like iron and calcium from the tofu, and antioxidants from the mushrooms and greens.

Cooking Time:

- Preparation time: 10 minutes
- Cook time: 15 minutes
- Total time: 25 minutes

Rating: ★★★★★

This Spicy Tofu and Mushroom Bowl is a flavorful and nutritious meal that's perfect for a quick dinner. Combining the hearty textures of tofu and mushrooms with the wholesomeness of brown rice or quinoa, this bowl is a powerhouse of protein and fiber. The spicy sauce adds a delightful kick, making it an excellent choice for those who enjoy a bit of heat with their meal. Easy to make and packed with health benefits, it's sure to satisfy both your taste buds and your nutritional needs.

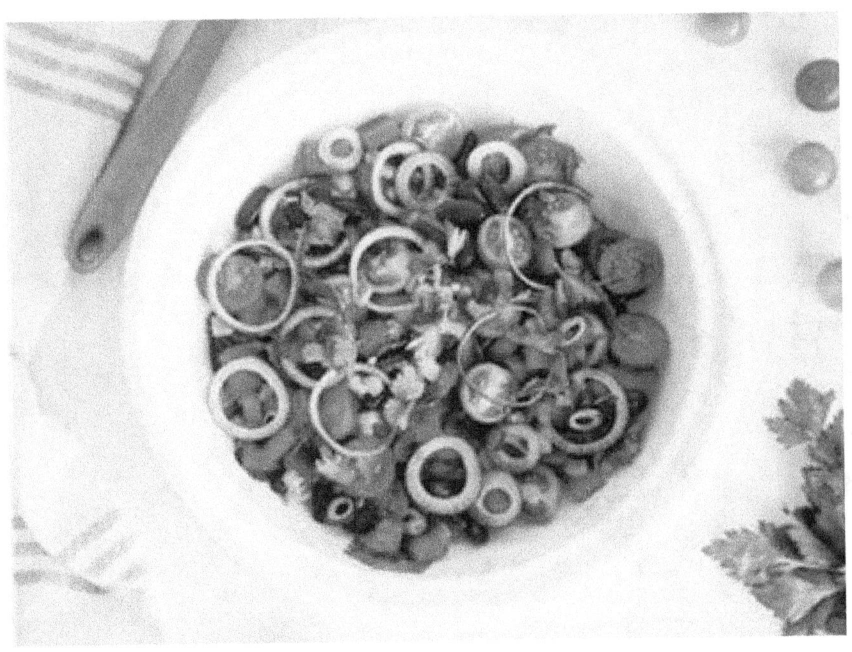

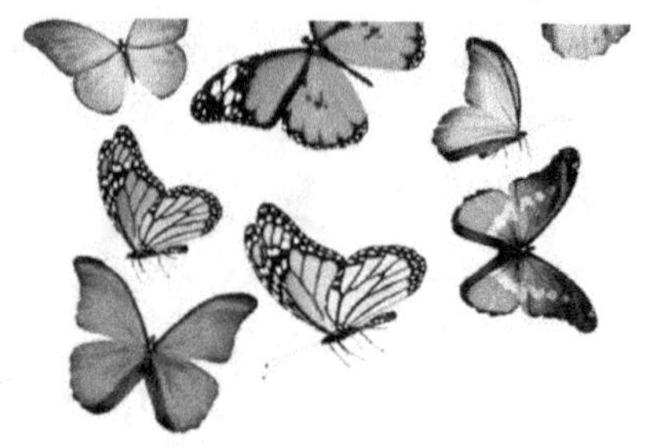

Starting a path to manage fibromyalgia with diet is a significant step in regaining your health and well-being. Each meal is an opportunity to fuel your body and alleviate your problems. Remember that growth happens one choice at a time. Be patient and gentle to yourself, and appreciate your minor achievements. Your efforts are not only altering your diet; they are also improving your life. You are not alone on this path. Keep going!

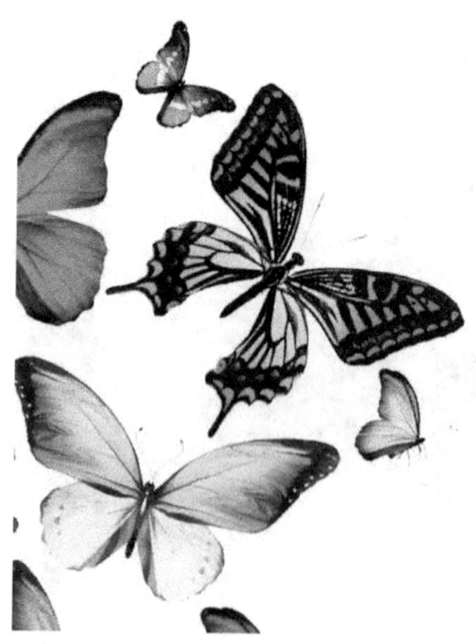

Chapter 4: Snacks and Sides

In our journey towards better health, especially for those managing fibromyalgia, snacks and sides play a pivotal role in maintaining energy and providing essential nutrients between main meals. This section is dedicated to quick, wholesome, and delicious recipes that can be prepared in 30 minutes or less. Perfect for any time of the day, these recipes ensure you're never far from a nutritious, anti-inflammatory snack or side that supports your overall well-being.

Cucumber and Hummus Bites

Ingredients:

- 1 large cucumber, sliced into rounds

- 1 cup prepared hummus (choose your favorite flavor)
- Paprika or smoked paprika for garnish
- Optional toppings: chopped parsley, sliced olives, or cherry tomato halves

Preparation:

1. Wash the cucumber and slice it into rounds, about 1/4 inch thick.
2. Spoon about a teaspoon of hummus onto each cucumber slice. Use a small spoon or piping bag for a neater presentation.
3. Sprinkle a little paprika over the hummus for color and flavor. If using, add your choice of optional toppings like chopped parsley, sliced olives, or cherry tomato halves for extra taste and visual appeal.
4. Arrange the cucumber and hummus bites on a platter and serve immediately, or chill in the refrigerator for a few minutes before serving if you prefer them cold.

Nutritional Value (per serving, about 5 bites):

- Calories: Approximately 100 kcal
- Protein: 3g
- Fat: 5g (healthy fats from hummus)
- Carbohydrates: 12g
- Fiber: 3g
- These bites are a low-calorie, nutritious snack that provides fiber from the cucumbers and protein from the hummus, making

them an excellent choice for a healthy, satisfying snack.

Cooking Time:

- Preparation time: 10 minutes
- Total time: 10 minutes

Rating: ★★★★★

Cucumber and Hummus Bites are the perfect quick and healthy snack or side dish. They're incredibly easy to make, requiring no cooking and less than 10 minutes of preparation time. This dish is not only nutritious and light but also versatile, allowing for various toppings to suit your taste. Ideal for anyone looking for a refreshing, guilt-free snack that's both delicious and beneficial for health, especially for those managing dietary concerns like fibromyalgia.

Sweet Potato and Kale Chips

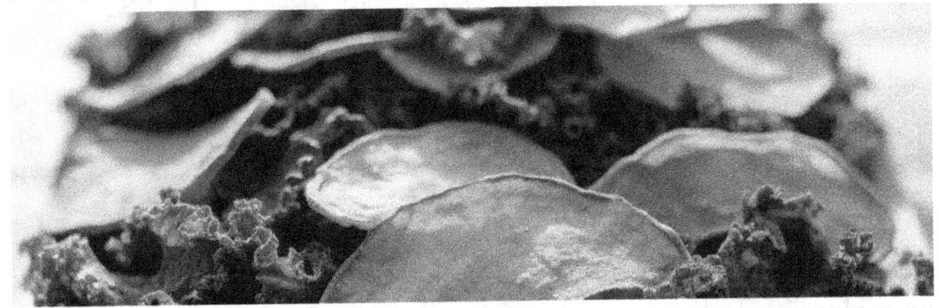

Ingredients:

- 1 large sweet potato, thinly sliced
- 2 cups kale leaves, torn into bite-sized pieces
- 2 tablespoons olive oil, divided
- Salt and pepper to taste
- Optional seasonings: paprika, garlic powder, or chili powder

Preparation:

1. Preheat your oven to 375°F (190°C). Line two baking sheets with parchment paper.

2. In a bowl, toss the sweet potato slices with 1 tablespoon of olive oil and a pinch of salt (and optional seasonings if you like). Spread the slices in a single layer on one of the prepared baking sheets.

3. In another bowl, toss the kale leaves with the remaining tablespoon of olive oil and a pinch of salt. Spread the kale leaves on the second baking sheet, ensuring they are not overlapping.

4. Bake the sweet potato slices for about 20-25 minutes, turning halfway through, until they are crispy and lightly browned.

5. Bake the kale chips for about 10-15 minutes, watching closely to prevent burning, until crispy.

6. Season both the sweet potato and kale chips with additional salt and pepper to taste. Let them cool on the baking sheets for a few minutes before serving.

Nutritional Value (per serving):

- Calories: Approximately 150 kcal
- Protein: 2g
- Fat: 7g (healthy fats from olive oil)
- Carbohydrates: 20g
- Fiber: 3g
- These chips offer a good source of vitamins A and C, calcium, and potassium. They're a healthier alternative to traditional chips, providing antioxidants and anti-inflammatory benefits.

Cooking Time:

- Preparation time: 10 minutes
- Cook time: 20-25 minutes for sweet potatoes, 10-15 minutes for kale
- Total time: 30-35 minutes

Rating: ★★★★★

Sweet Potato and Kale Chips are a delicious, easy-to-make snack that's both nutritious and satisfying. Perfect for those looking for a healthy, crunchy treat, these chips are a fantastic way to enjoy the flavors and benefits of sweet potatoes and kale in a fun, snackable form. Whether you're craving something salty or just need a quick side dish, these chips are sure to hit the spot while supporting your health goals.

Almond and Flaxseed Energy Balls

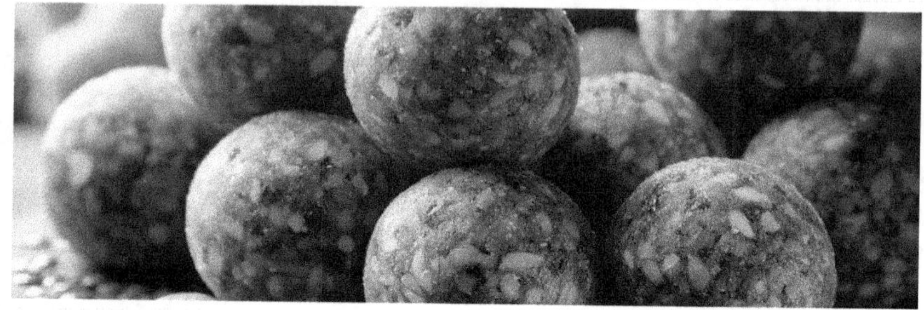

Ingredients:

- 1 cup almonds
- 1/2 cup flaxseed meal
- 1/3 cup rolled oats (choose gluten-free if needed)
- 1/4 cup honey or maple syrup (for a vegan alternative)
- 1/2 cup natural peanut butter or almond butter
- 1 teaspoon vanilla extract
- Optional: 1/4 cup mini chocolate chips or dried fruit

Quick Preparation:

1. Place almonds in a food processor and pulse until they are finely chopped, not into a flour, to maintain texture.
2. In a large bowl, mix the chopped almonds, flaxseed meal, and rolled oats.

3. Warm the honey (or maple syrup) and peanut butter (or almond butter) in a microwave for about 20-30 seconds. This helps in mixing them easily.

4. Pour the honey (or maple syrup) and peanut butter (or almond butter) mixture into the dry ingredients. Add vanilla extract. Stir until all components are fully combined. The mixture should be sticky. If it's too dry, add a bit more honey or peanut butter.

5. If using, fold in mini chocolate chips or dried fruit.

6. With damp hands, form the mixture into small balls, about 1 inch in diameter.

7. Place the energy balls on a plate or tray lined with parchment paper. They can be enjoyed immediately or stored in the refrigerator to firm up a bit, though chilling is optional based on preference.

Nutritional Value (approximate per ball, for 20 balls total):

- Calories: 150 kcal
- Protein: 4g
- Fat: 9g
- Carbohydrates: 12g
- Fiber: 3g

Total Time:

- 15 minutes (with no need for chilling unless preferred)

Rating: ★★★★★

These Quick Almond and Flaxseed Energy Balls are an ideal snack for those short on time but looking for a nutritious, energy-boosting treat. Easy to make and requiring no baking, they're perfect for a healthy snack that combines the nutritional benefits of almonds, flaxseed, and oats into a delicious bite-sized ball.

Quinoa Tabbouleh

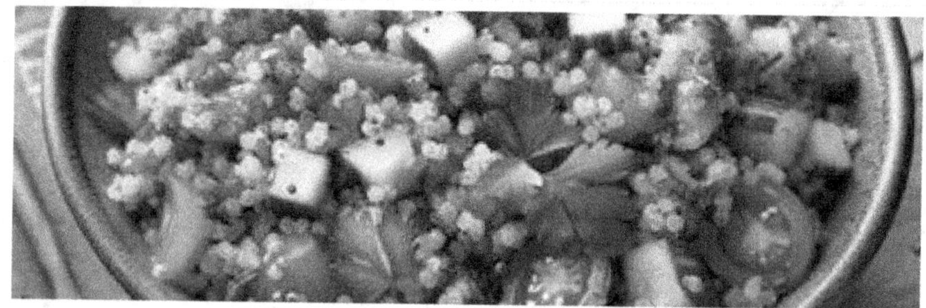

Ingredients:

- 1 cup quinoa, rinsed
- 2 cups water
- 1 cup fresh parsley, finely chopped
- 1/2 cup fresh mint, finely chopped
- 1/2 cup cucumber, diced
- 1/2 cup cherry tomatoes, halved
- 1/4 cup red onion, finely diced
- 3 tablespoons olive oil
- 2 tablespoons lemon juice
- Salt and pepper to taste

Preparation:

1. In a medium saucepan, bring the 2 cups of water to a boil. Add the rinsed quinoa and reduce the heat to low. Cover and simmer

for about 15 minutes, or until the quinoa is cooked and the water is absorbed. Fluff the quinoa with a fork and allow it to cool slightly.

2. In a large bowl, combine the cooled quinoa with the parsley, mint, cucumber, cherry tomatoes, and red onion.

3. In a small bowl, whisk together the olive oil and lemon juice, adding salt and pepper to taste. Pour this dressing over the quinoa mixture and toss until everything is evenly coated.

4. Adjust seasoning with more salt, pepper, or lemon juice according to your preference.

5. Let the tabbouleh sit for a few minutes to allow the flavors to meld together before serving.

Nutritional Value (per serving):

- Calories: Approximately 200 kcal
- Protein: 6g
- Fat: 9g (healthy fats from olive oil)
- Carbohydrates: 27g
- Fiber: 5g

- This dish is rich in vitamins A and C from the parsley and tomatoes, and provides a good source of plant-based protein and fiber from the quinoa.

Cooking Time:

- Preparation time: 10 minutes
- Cook time: 15 minutes
- Total time: 25 minutes

Rating: ★★★★★

Quinoa Tabbouleh is a refreshing, nutritious salad perfect for a quick and healthy meal or side dish. With its combination of fresh herbs, vegetables, and the protein-packed quinoa, this dish is a delightful twist on traditional tabbouleh. It's easy to prepare, making it an excellent choice for those looking for a wholesome, flavorful option that supports a healthy lifestyle, especially when time is limited.

Baked Zucchini Fries

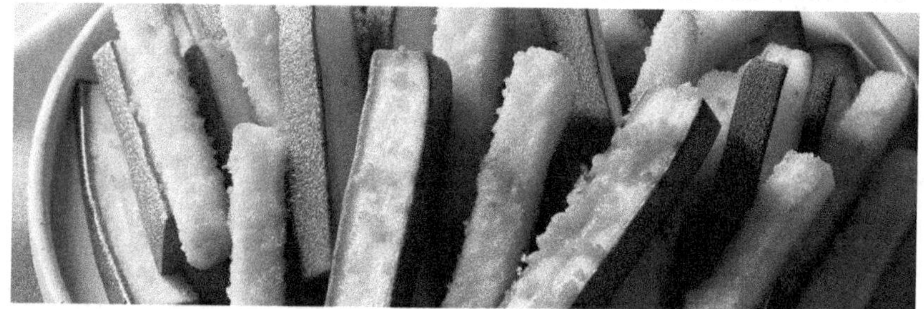

Ingredients:

- 2 medium zucchinis
- 1/2 cup grated Parmesan cheese
- 1/2 cup breadcrumbs (use gluten-free breadcrumbs for a gluten-free option)
- 1 teaspoon garlic powder
- 1 teaspoon Italian seasoning
- Salt and pepper to taste
- 2 eggs, beaten

Preparation:

1. Preheat your oven to 425°F (220°C). Line a baking sheet with parchment paper or lightly grease it.
2. Cut the zucchinis into fries-sized sticks.
3. In a shallow dish, mix together the grated Parmesan cheese, breadcrumbs, garlic powder, Italian seasoning, salt, and pepper.
4. In another shallow dish, beat the eggs.
5. Dip each zucchini stick into the beaten eggs, then coat it in the breadcrumb mixture. Place the coated zucchini fries on the prepared baking sheet.
6. Bake in the preheated oven for about 20 minutes, or until the zucchini fries are golden and crispy. Flip the fries halfway through the baking time to ensure even crispiness.
7. Serve immediately, optionally with a side of marinara sauce for dipping.

Nutritional Value (per serving, serves 4):

- Calories: Approximately 150 kcal
- Protein: 8g
- Fat: 7g
- Carbohydrates: 15g
- Fiber: 2g
- Zucchini fries offer a healthier alternative to traditional fries, providing vitamins A and C, calcium from the Parmesan, and a good balance of protein and fiber.

Cooking Time:

- Preparation time: 10 minutes
- Cook time: 20 minutes
- Total time: 30 minutes

Rating: ★★★★★

These Baked Zucchini Fries are a crunchy, delicious snack or side dish that's easy to make and perfect for anyone looking for a healthier alternative to traditional fries. With a crispy Parmesan and breadcrumb coating seasoned with Italian herbs, they're packed with flavor and provide a nutritious way to enjoy zucchini. Ideal for a quick, satisfying treat that fits well into a balanced diet.

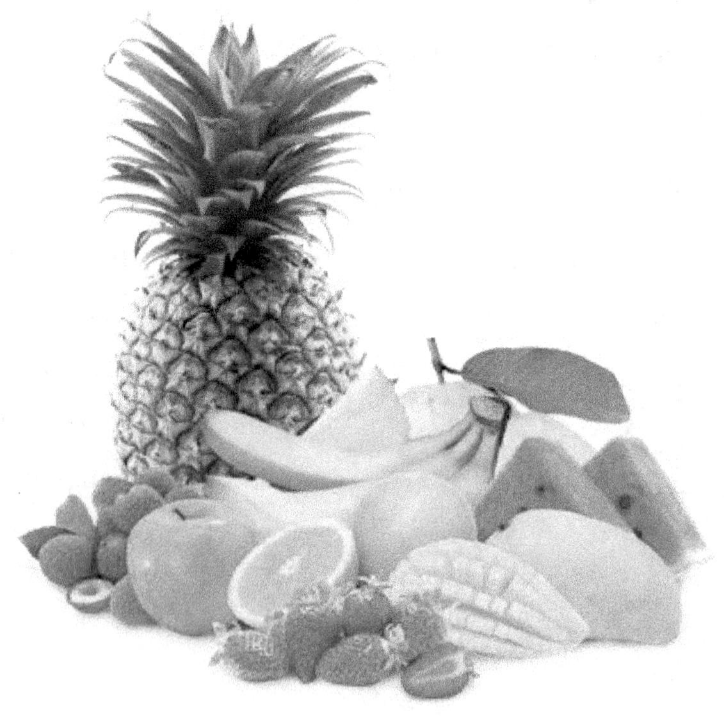

Chapter 5: Seafoods and Fish

Dive into the delightful world of seafood and fish, where each recipe is designed to bring the ocean's bounty right to your table in 30 minutes or less. This chapter is dedicated to those who seek not only to nourish their bodies but also to enjoy the exquisite flavors that only seafood can offer. Perfect for individuals managing fibromyalgia, our collection features dishes rich in omega-3 fatty acids, known for their anti-inflammatory properties and health benefits. From the simplicity of baked cod to the robust flavors of spicy shrimp tacos, these recipes are crafted to provide a quick, nutritious, and delicious meal option for any day of the week. Whether you're a seasoned seafood lover or just starting to explore the vast sea of options, this chapter promises a hassle-free cooking experience that doesn't compromise on taste or nutritional value.

Pan-Seared Scallops with Lemon Butter Sauce

Ingredients:

- 1-pound large sea scallops, patted dry
- Salt and pepper to taste
- 2 tablespoons olive oil

- 2 tablespoons unsalted butter
- 1 clove garlic, minced
- Juice of 1 lemon
- 1 tablespoon fresh parsley, chopped
- Additional parsley and lemon wedges for garnish

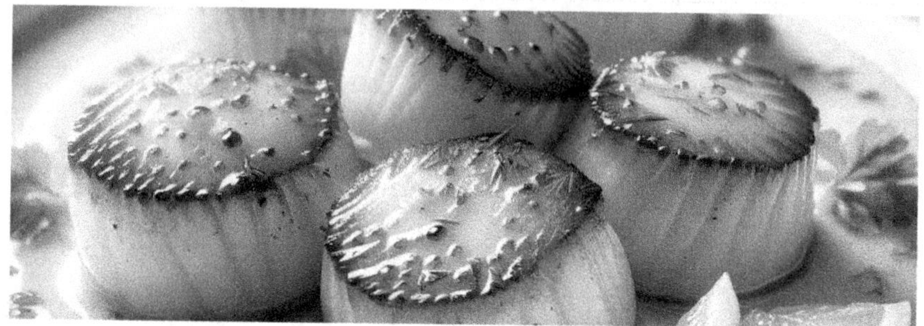

Preparation:

1. Season the scallops with salt and pepper on both sides.

2. Heat the olive oil in a large skillet over medium-high heat. Once hot, add the scallops, making sure not to overcrowd the pan. Sear for about 2 minutes on each side or until a golden crust forms and they are just cooked through. Remove the scallops from the skillet and set aside.

3. In the same skillet, reduce the heat to medium. Add the butter and garlic, sautéing for about 1 minute until the garlic is fragrant but not browned.

4. Stir in the lemon juice and chopped parsley, scraping up any browned bits from the bottom of the pan. Cook for another minute until the sauce has slightly thickened.

5. Return the scallops to the pan, spooning the sauce over them to warm through.
6. Serve immediately, garnished with additional parsley and lemon wedges on the side.

Nutritional Value (per serving, serves 4):

- Calories: Approximately 200 kcal
- Protein: 14g
- Fat: 15g (healthy fats from olive oil and unsaturated fats from butter)
- Carbohydrates: 3g
- Fiber: 0g
- Scallops are a great source of lean protein and provide important nutrients such as vitamin B12 and omega-3 fatty acids, which are beneficial for heart health and reducing inflammation.

Cooking Time:

- Preparation time: 5 minutes
- Cook time: 10 minutes
- Total time: 15 minutes

Rating: ★★★★★

Pan-Seared Scallops with Lemon Butter Sauce is an elegant, flavorful dish that can elevate any meal to a restaurant-quality experience. Despite its luxurious taste, it's surprisingly quick and easy to prepare, making it perfect for a nutritious weeknight dinner or a special occasion. This recipe beautifully showcases the delicate texture and sweet flavor of scallops, complemented by the bright, tangy sauce.

Quick Spicy Salmon Tacos

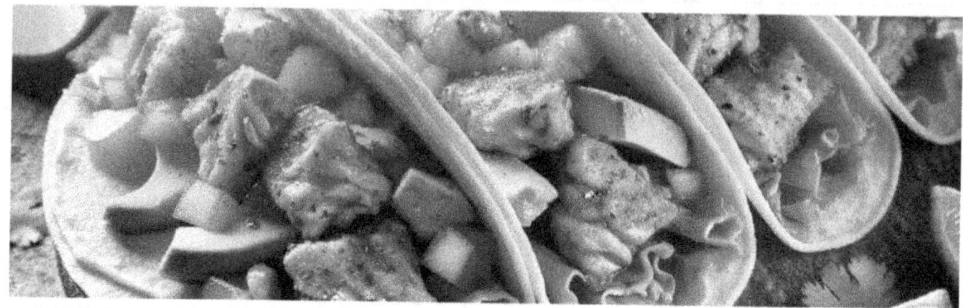

Ingredients:

- 1 pound salmon fillet, skin removed
- 1 tablespoon olive oil
- 1 tablespoon chili powder
- 1 teaspoon cumin
- 1/2 teaspoon smoked paprika
- Salt and pepper to taste
- 8 small corn tortillas
- 1/2 cup cabbage, thinly sliced
- 1 avocado, sliced
- 1/4 cup fresh cilantro, chopped
- Lime wedges, for serving
- Optional: sour cream or Greek yogurt, and hot sauce for topping

Preparation:

1. Preheat your oven to 400°F (200°C) or heat a grill to medium-high.

2. Mix the chili powder, cumin, smoked paprika, salt, and pepper together in a small bowl. Rub the salmon fillet with olive oil and then evenly coat with the spice mixture.

3. Place the salmon on a baking sheet lined with parchment paper (if baking) and cook in the preheated oven for 12-15 minutes, or until the salmon is cooked through and flakes easily with a fork. If grilling, place the salmon on the grill and cook for about 3-5 minutes per side.

4. While the salmon is cooking, warm the corn tortillas in the oven or on the grill for about 1 minute on each side.

5. Once the salmon is done, use a fork to flake it into pieces.

6. Assemble the tacos by dividing the flaked salmon among the warmed tortillas. Top with sliced cabbage, avocado slices, and chopped cilantro. Serve with lime wedges on the side, and if desired, a dollop of sour cream or Greek yogurt and a drizzle of hot sauce.

Nutritional Value (per serving, 2 tacos):

- Calories: Approximately 350 kcal
- Protein: 23g
- Fat: 20g (healthy fats from salmon and avocado)
- Carbohydrates: 22g
- Fiber: 5g

Cooking Time:

- Preparation time: 10 minutes
- Cook time: 15 minutes
- Total time: 25 minutes

Rating: ★★★★★

Quick Spicy Salmon Tacos are a delicious, nutritious twist on traditional tacos, offering a perfect balance of flavors and textures. This dish combines the heart-healthy benefits of salmon with the freshness of avocado and cilantro, all wrapped up in a soft corn tortilla. It's an ideal meal for anyone looking for a quick, flavorful, and health-conscious option that can be prepared in less than 30 minutes.

Shrimp Avocado Mango Salad

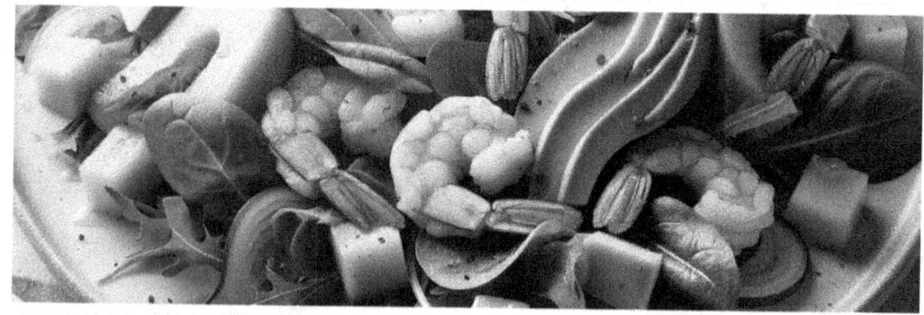

Ingredients:

- 1-pound cooked shrimp, peeled and deveined
- 1 ripe avocado, diced
- 1 ripe mango, diced
- 1/2 red onion, finely chopped
- 1/4 cup fresh cilantro, chopped
- Juice of 1 lime

- 2 tablespoons olive oil
- Salt and pepper to taste
- Optional: mixed greens or baby spinach for serving

Preparation:

1. In a large bowl, combine the cooked shrimp, diced avocado, diced mango, finely chopped red onion, and chopped cilantro.
2. In a small bowl, whisk together the lime juice, olive oil, salt, and pepper to create the dressing.
3. Pour the dressing over the shrimp mixture and gently toss to ensure everything is evenly coated.
4. If desired, serve the salad over a bed of mixed greens or baby spinach for added nutrients and color.
5. Adjust seasoning with additional salt, pepper, or lime juice according to your taste.

Nutritional Value (per serving, serves 4):

- Calories: Approximately 250 kcal
- Protein: 24g
- Fat: 12g (healthy fats from avocado and olive oil)
- Carbohydrates: 15g
- Fiber: 3g

Cooking Time:

- Preparation time: 15 minutes
- Total time: 15 minutes

Rating: ★★★★★

Shrimp Avocado Mango Salad is a vibrant, refreshing dish perfect for a quick, nutritious meal. It combines the sweetness of mango with the creaminess of avocado and the savory taste of shrimp, all brought together with a zesty lime dressing. This salad is not only a feast for the eyes but also packed with nutrients, making it an excellent choice for those seeking a healthy, flavorful option that's easy to prepare. Ideal for a light lunch, dinner, or as a side, this dish is sure to delight anyone looking for a delicious, health-conscious meal in 30 minutes or less.

Tilapia with Mango Salsa

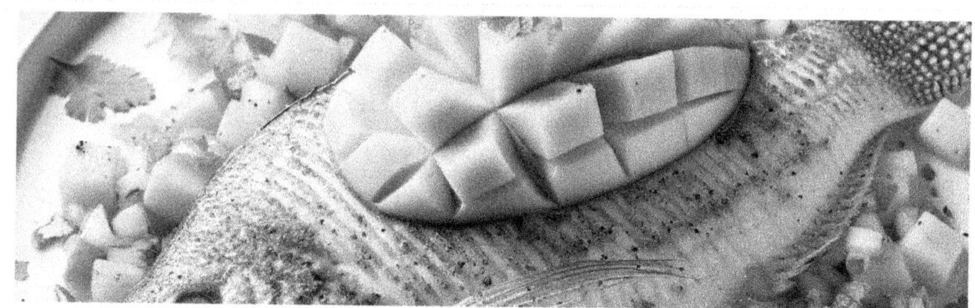

Ingredients:

- 4 tilapia fillets
- Salt and pepper to taste
- 2 tablespoons olive oil

For the Mango Salsa:

- 1 ripe mango, diced
- 1/2 red bell pepper, diced
- 1/4 cup red onion, finely chopped

- 1/4 cup fresh cilantro, chopped
- Juice of 1 lime
- Salt to taste

Preparation:

1. Season the tilapia fillets with salt and pepper on both sides.
2. Heat olive oil in a large skillet over medium-high heat. Once hot, add the tilapia fillets and cook for about 3-4 minutes on each side, or until the fish flakes easily with a fork and is lightly golden.
3. While the tilapia is cooking, prepare the mango salsa by combining the diced mango, red bell pepper, red onion, cilantro, and lime juice in a bowl. Season with salt to taste and mix well.
4. Once the tilapia is cooked, remove from heat and let it rest for a minute.
5. Serve the tilapia topped with a generous portion of the mango salsa.

Nutritional Value (per serving):

- Calories: Approximately 250 kcal
- Protein: 23g
- Fat: 10g (healthy fats from olive oil)
- Carbohydrates: 15g
- Fiber: 2g

Cooking Time:

- Preparation time: 10 minutes
- Cook time: 8 minutes
- Total time: 18 minutes

Rating: ★★★★★

Tilapia with Mango Salsa is a light, flavorful dish that embodies the essence of quick and healthy cooking. The freshness of the mango salsa complements the mild taste of tilapia, creating a meal that's both nutritious and delightful. This dish is perfect for those seeking a quick, delicious, and healthy option that can be prepared in under 30 minutes, making it an ideal choice for busy weeknights or a special, hassle-free dinner.

Garlic Lemon Tuna Patties

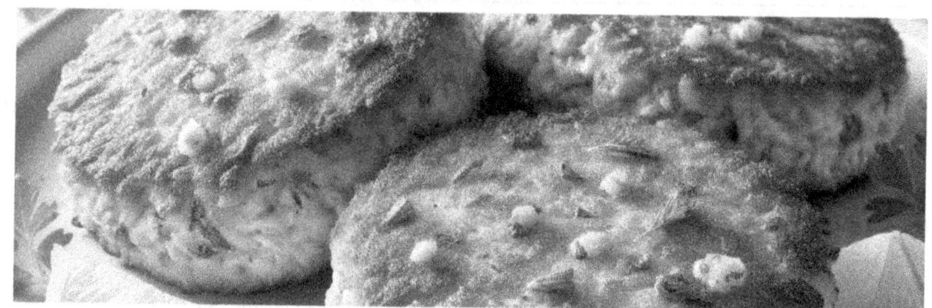

Ingredients:

- 2 cans (5 oz each) tuna in water, drained
- 1/4 cup breadcrumbs (use gluten-free breadcrumbs for a gluten-free option)
- 1 large egg
- 2 tablespoons mayonnaise
- 2 cloves garlic, minced
- Zest and juice of 1 lemon

- 2 tablespoons fresh parsley, chopped
- Salt and pepper to taste
- 2 tablespoons olive oil for frying

Preparation:

1. In a large bowl, combine the drained tuna, breadcrumbs, egg, mayonnaise, minced garlic, lemon zest, lemon juice, and chopped parsley. Season with salt and pepper to taste. Mix well until the ingredients are evenly distributed.
2. Form the mixture into patties, about 1/2 inch thick.
3. Heat olive oil in a large skillet over medium heat. Once hot, add the tuna patties. Cook for about 3-4 minutes on each side, or until they are golden brown and crispy.
4. Serve the patties warm, optionally with a side of mixed greens or your favorite dipping sauce.

Nutritional Value (per serving, based on 4 servings):

- Calories: Approximately 200 kcal
- Protein: 20g
- Fat: 10g (healthy fats from olive oil and mayonnaise)
- Carbohydrates: 5g
- Fiber: 0.5g

Cooking Time:

- Preparation time: 10 minutes
- Cook time: 8 minutes
- Total time: 18 minutes

Rating: ★★★★★

Garlic Lemon Tuna Patties are a delicious, quick, and easy meal perfect for any time of the day. They offer a fantastic way to enjoy the health benefits of tuna, packed with protein and omega-3 fatty acids, in a flavorful and convenient form. The addition of lemon and garlic adds a fresh and zesty taste that elevates this dish beyond the ordinary. Ready in under 30 minutes, these patties are ideal for a nutritious and satisfying meal that fits into any busy schedule.

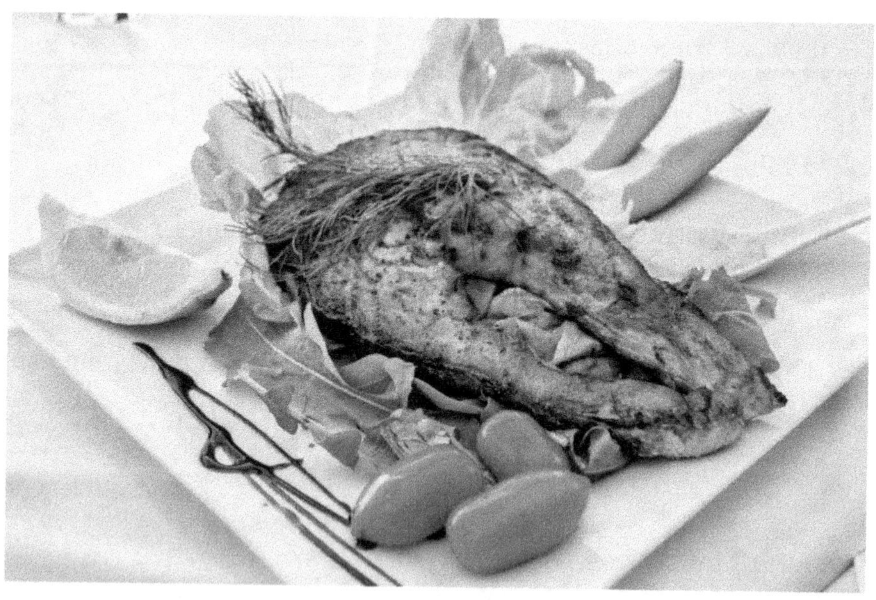

Chapter 6: Meat and Poultry

This chapter offers a selection of meat and poultry recipes designed for those managing fibromyalgia, focusing on lean proteins and anti-inflammatory ingredients. Each dish, ready in 30 minutes or less, is crafted to support muscle health and energy without sacrificing flavor. We aim to provide nutritious, easy-to-prepare meals that fit into a fibromyalgia-friendly diet. Whether you're looking for a quick weeknight dinner or a healthy meal option, these recipes are sure to satisfy your cravings and nutritional needs efficiently.

Turkey and Spinach Meatballs

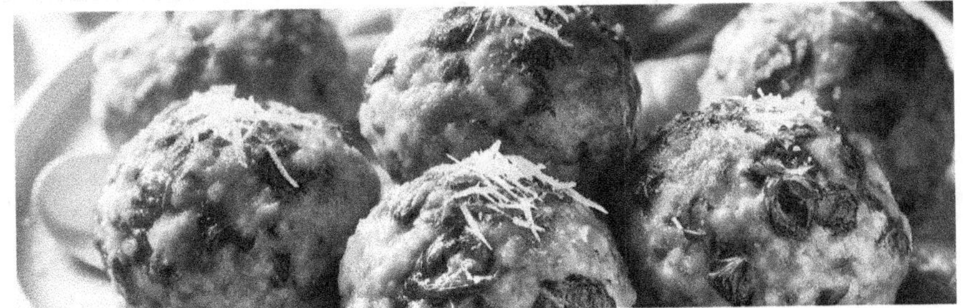

Ingredients:

- 1 pound ground turkey

- 1 cup fresh spinach, finely chopped
- 1/2 cup breadcrumbs (use gluten-free breadcrumbs for a gluten-free option)
- 1/4 cup Parmesan cheese, grated
- 1 large egg
- 2 cloves garlic, minced
- 1 teaspoon dried oregano
- Salt and pepper to taste
- 1 tablespoon olive oil, for cooking

Preparation:

1. In a large bowl, combine the ground turkey, finely chopped spinach, breadcrumbs, grated Parmesan cheese, egg, minced garlic, dried oregano, salt, and pepper. Mix until well combined.
2. Form the mixture into small, round meatballs, about 1 inch in diameter.
3. Heat the olive oil in a large skillet over medium heat. Once hot, add the meatballs to the skillet, cooking in batches if necessary to avoid overcrowding. Cook for about 5-7 minutes, turning occasionally, until the meatballs are golden on all sides and cooked through.
4. Serve the turkey and spinach meatballs hot, optionally with your favorite sauce or as part of a meal with vegetables or whole grains.

Nutritional Value (per serving, based on 4 servings):

- Calories: Approximately 220 kcal
- Protein: 27g
- Fat: 10g (healthy fats from olive oil and Parmesan)
- Carbohydrates: 9g
- Fiber: 1g

Cooking Time:

- Preparation time: 10 minutes
- Cook time: 10 minutes
- Total time: 20 minutes

Rating: ★★★★★

Turkey and Spinach Meatballs are a delicious, easy-to-make option for a healthy, satisfying meal. They're perfect for those looking to include more lean proteins and vegetables in their diet. The combination of turkey and spinach not only makes these meatballs tender and flavorful but also boosts their nutritional profile, making them a fantastic choice for anyone, especially those managing conditions like fibromyalgia.

Chicken and Quinoa Soup

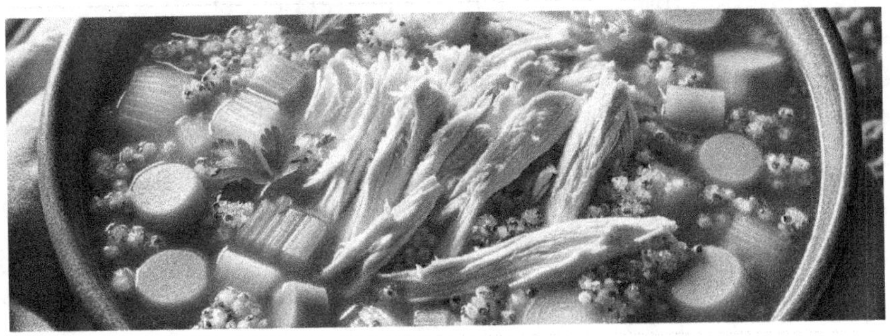

Ingredients:

- 2 tablespoons olive oil
- 1 medium onion, diced
- 2 carrots, peeled and diced
- 2 stalks celery, diced
- 2 cloves garlic, minced
- 1/2-pound chicken breast, cut into small pieces
- 4 cups chicken broth
- 1/2 cup quinoa, rinsed
- 1 teaspoon dried thyme
- Salt and pepper to taste
- 2 cups baby spinach leaves
- Lemon wedges, for serving

Preparation:

1. Heat olive oil in a large pot over medium heat. Add the diced onion, carrots, and celery. Sauté for about 5 minutes until the vegetables start to soften.

2. Add the minced garlic and chicken pieces to the pot. Cook, stirring occasionally, until the chicken is no longer pink on the outside, about 5 minutes.

3. Pour in the chicken broth and bring the mixture to a boil. Stir in the rinsed quinoa, dried thyme, salt, and pepper.

4. Reduce heat to a simmer, cover, and cook for about 15 minutes, or until the quinoa is fully cooked and the chicken is tender.

5. Stir in the baby spinach and cook until just wilted, about 1-2 minutes.

6. Serve the soup hot with lemon wedges on the side for squeezing.

Nutritional Value (per serving, serves 4):

- Calories: Approximately 250 kcal
- Protein: 20g
- Fat: 8g (healthy fats from olive oil)
- Carbohydrates: 23g
- Fiber: 4g

Cooking Time:

- Preparation time: 5 minutes
- Cook time: 25 minutes
- Total time: 30 minutes

Rating: ★★★★★

Chicken and Quinoa Soup is a hearty, nutritious meal that comes together quickly, making it perfect for a healthy dinner on busy nights. Packed with lean protein, whole grains, and vegetables, this soup is designed to satisfy hunger while providing essential nutrients. It's an excellent choice for anyone looking for a comforting, easy-to-make dish that supports a healthy lifestyle, especially those managing fibromyalgia with diet.

Balsamic Glazed Steak Rolls

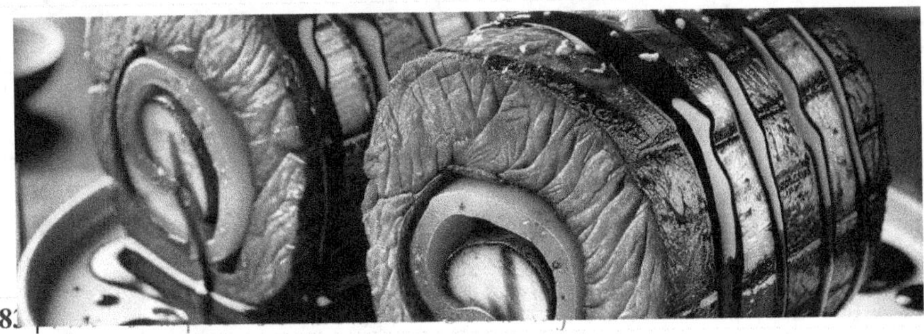

Ingredients:

- 1 pound flank steak, thinly sliced into strips
- Salt and pepper to taste
- 2 tablespoons olive oil, divided
- 1 red bell pepper, thinly sliced
- 1 zucchini, thinly sliced
- 1 carrot, thinly sliced
- 1/2 onion, thinly sliced
- 2 cloves garlic, minced
- 1/4 cup balsamic vinegar
- 2 tablespoons soy sauce (or tamari for a gluten-free option)
- 1 tablespoon honey
- Fresh parsley, chopped, for garnish

Preparation:

1. Season the flank steak strips with salt and pepper.
2. Heat 1 tablespoon of olive oil in a large skillet over medium-high heat. Quickly sauté the vegetables (bell pepper, zucchini, carrot, and onion) until just tender but still crisp, about 2-3 minutes. Add the garlic in the last 30 seconds. Remove from heat and set aside.
3. Lay out the steak strips and place a small amount of the vegetable mixture at one end of each strip. Roll up the steak around the vegetables and secure with a toothpick.

4. In the same skillet, heat the remaining tablespoon of olive oil over medium-high heat. Add the steak rolls, seam-side down, and cook for about 2-3 minutes per side, or until browned to your liking.

5. In a small bowl, whisk together the balsamic vinegar, soy sauce, and honey. Pour this glaze over the steak rolls in the skillet, turning them to coat evenly. Cook for an additional 1-2 minutes, until the glaze has thickened slightly.

6. Serve the steak rolls garnished with fresh parsley and drizzled with any remaining glaze from the skillet.

Nutritional Value (per serving, serves 4):

- Calories: Approximately 300 kcal
- Protein: 25g
- Fat: 15g (healthy fats from olive oil)
- Carbohydrates: 15g
- Fiber: 2g

Cooking Time:

- Preparation time: 10 minutes
- Cook time: 15 minutes
- Total time: 25 minutes

Rating: ★★★★★

Balsamic Glazed Steak Rolls are a visually appealing and flavor-packed dish that's perfect for a quick and nutritious meal. The combination of tender steak, crisp vegetables, and a sweet and tangy balsamic glaze offers a gourmet experience that's easy to achieve in under 30 minutes. This recipe is ideal for those looking to impress with a delicious and healthy dish, especially suitable for managing a balanced diet.

Quick Chicken Parmesan

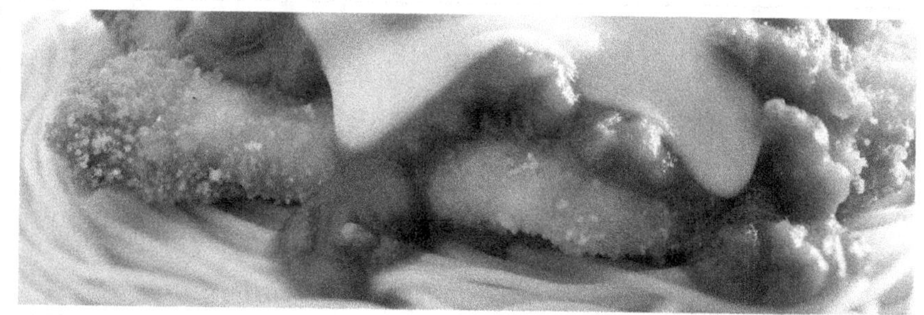

Ingredients:

- 4 boneless, skinless chicken breasts, pounded to even thickness
- Salt and pepper to taste
- 1/2 cup all-purpose flour (use gluten-free flour for a gluten-free option)
- 2 large eggs, beaten
- 1 cup breadcrumbs (use gluten-free breadcrumbs for a gluten-free option)
- 1/2 cup grated Parmesan cheese
- 2 tablespoons olive oil
- 1 cup marinara sauce
- 1 cup shredded mozzarella cheese
- Fresh basil leaves for garnish

Preparation:

1. Preheat your oven to 400°F (200°C).
2. Season the chicken breasts with salt and pepper. Dredge each chicken breast first in flour, shaking off the excess, then dip in beaten eggs, and finally coat with a mixture of breadcrumbs and grated Parmesan cheese.
3. Heat olive oil in a large oven-proof skillet over medium-high heat. Add the chicken and cook for 2-3 minutes on each side, or until golden brown.
4. Pour the marinara sauce over the chicken in the skillet. Sprinkle shredded mozzarella cheese on top of each chicken breast.
5. Transfer the skillet to the preheated oven and bake for about 10-15 minutes, or until the chicken is cooked through and the cheese is melted and bubbly.
6. Garnish with fresh basil leaves before serving.

Nutritional Value (per serving, serves 4):

- Calories: Approximately 450 kcal
- Protein: 38g
- Fat: 20g (healthy fats from olive oil)
- Carbohydrates: 30g (if using gluten-free options, carbs may vary)
- Fiber: 2g
- This dish is a good source of high-quality protein from chicken, calcium

from the cheese, and provides antioxidants from the marinara sauce.

Cooking Time:

- Preparation time: 10 minutes
- Cook time: 20 minutes
- Total time: 30 minutes

Rating: ★★★★★

Quick Chicken Parmesan is a simplified version of the classic dish, offering all the comforting flavors and cheesy goodness in a fraction of the time. Perfect for a hearty dinner on busy nights, this recipe combines tender chicken with a rich tomato sauce and melted cheese, all baked to perfection. It's an easy, delicious way to enjoy a restaurant-quality meal at home, suitable for everyone in the family.

Spiced Lamb Chops with Yogurt Sauce

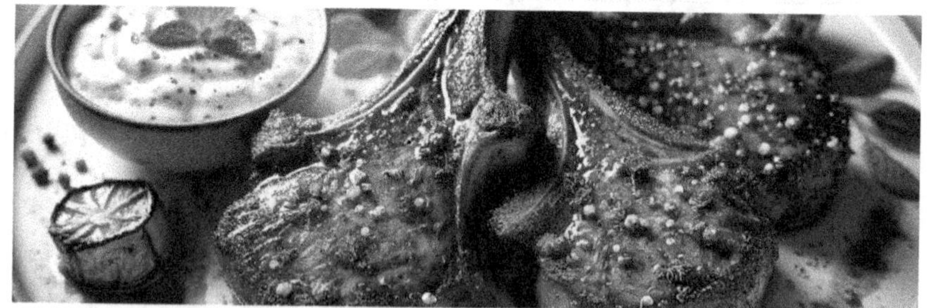

Ingredients:

- 8 lamb chops
- 2 tablespoons olive oil

- 1 teaspoon ground cumin
- 1 teaspoon smoked paprika
- 1/2 teaspoon garlic powder
- Salt and pepper to taste

For the Yogurt Sauce:

- 1 cup Greek yogurt
- 1 clove garlic, minced
- 1 tablespoon fresh mint, finely chopped
- Juice of 1/2 lemon
- Salt to taste

Preparation:

1. In a small bowl, mix together the ground cumin, smoked paprika, garlic powder, salt, and pepper. Rub this spice mixture over both sides of the lamb chops.
2. Heat olive oil in a large skillet over medium-high heat. Add the lamb chops and cook for about 3-4 minutes on each side for medium-rare, or longer to your desired doneness.
3. While the lamb chops are cooking, prepare the yogurt sauce by combining Greek yogurt, minced garlic, chopped mint, lemon juice, and salt in a bowl. Mix well until smooth.
4. Once the lamb chops are cooked, remove them from the skillet and let them rest for a few minutes.
5. Serve the lamb chops with a dollop of the yogurt sauce on top or on the side for dipping.

Nutritional Value (per serving, serves 4):

- Calories: Approximately 350 kcal
- Protein: 25g
- Fat: 25g (healthy fats from olive oil and lamb)
- Carbohydrates: 4g
- Fiber: 0g

- The lamb chops are a great source of high-quality protein and essential nutrients, while the yogurt sauce adds a refreshing touch and provides calcium and probiotics.

Cooking Time:

- Preparation time: 10 minutes
- Cook time: 8 minutes
- Total time: 18 minutes

Rating: ★★★★★

Spiced Lamb Chops with Yogurt Sauce is a quick and flavorful dish that brings a touch of elegance to your dining table in less than 30 minutes. The combination of warm spices on the lamb and the cool, creamy yogurt sauce creates a delightful contrast of flavors and textures. This dish is perfect for a special occasion or a gourmet weeknight dinner, offering a satisfying and nutritious meal that's easy to prepare and sure to impress.

Chapter 7: Desserts

In this chapter, we delve into the sweet finale of our meal journey, focusing on desserts that cater to the dietary needs of those managing fibromyalgia. Understanding the importance of maintaining a balanced and anti-inflammatory diet, we've curated a collection of dessert recipes that are not only quick to prepare, within 30 minutes or less, but also mindful of nutritional value. From the richness of avocado chocolate mousse to the natural sweetness of honey-roasted pears, each recipe is designed to satisfy your sweet tooth without overwhelming your system with processed sugars or unhealthy fats. These desserts are perfect for enjoying a guilt-free indulgence that complements your health-focused lifestyle, proving that you can still delight in the pleasures of sweet treats while adhering to a diet that supports your well-being.

Avocado Chocolate Mousse

Ingredients:

- 2 ripe avocados, peeled and pitted

- 1/4 cup cocoa powder, unsweetened

- 1/4 cup honey or maple syrup (for vegan option)
- 1/2 teaspoon vanilla extract
- A pinch of salt
- Optional for serving: fresh berries, whipped cream, or coconut cream

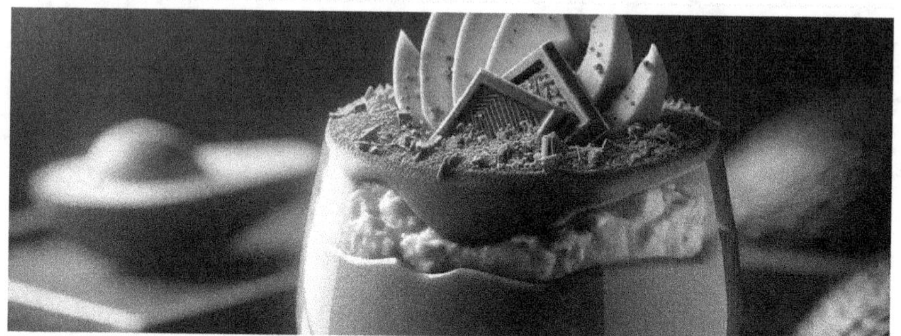

Preparation:

1. In a blender or food processor, combine the avocados, cocoa powder, honey (or maple syrup), vanilla extract, and a pinch of salt. Blend until the mixture is smooth and creamy, scraping down the sides as needed.

2. Taste the mousse and adjust the sweetness if necessary, adding a bit more honey or maple syrup if desired.

3. Divide the mousse into individual serving dishes and refrigerate for at least 15 minutes to chill and set slightly, making it more mousse-like in texture.

4. Serve chilled, garnished with fresh berries, whipped cream, or coconut cream if using.

Nutritional Value (per serving, serves 4):

- Calories: Approximately 230 kcal
- Protein: 3g
- Fat: 15g (healthy fats from avocado)
- Carbohydrates: 28g
- Fiber: 7g

- This dessert is rich in healthy fats, fiber, and antioxidants from the cocoa and avocados, making it a nutritious alternative to traditional chocolate mousse.

Cooking Time:

- Preparation time: 10 minutes
- Chill time: 15 minutes
- Total time: 25 minutes

Rating: ★★★★★

Avocado Chocolate Mousse is a decadent, creamy dessert that marries the nutritional powerhouse of avocados with the rich flavor of cocoa. This dessert not only satisfies the most intense chocolate cravings but does so in a health-conscious way, suitable for those managing fibromyalgia or anyone looking for a healthier dessert option. It's a perfect example of how quick, simple ingredients can be transformed into a luxurious treat in less than 30 minutes, making it ideal for a quick dessert that doesn't compromise on health or taste.

Coconut Flour Pancakes with Berry Compote

Ingredients:

For the Pancakes:

- 1/2 cup coconut flour
- 1 teaspoon baking powder
- 1/4 teaspoon salt
- 4 eggs
- 1 cup almond milk (or any milk of choice)
- 2 tablespoons honey or maple syrup
- 1 teaspoon vanilla extract
- Coconut oil or butter for cooking

For the Berry Compote:

- 2 cups mixed berries (fresh or frozen)
- 2 tablespoons honey or maple syrup
- Juice of 1/2 lemon

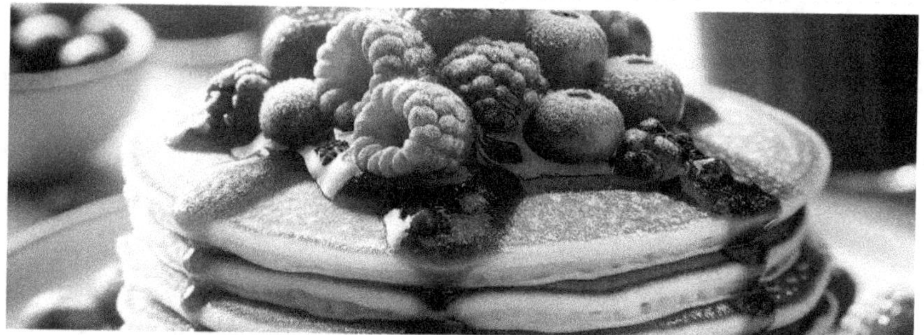

Preparation:

1. Pancakes: In a large bowl, whisk together coconut flour, baking powder, and salt. In another bowl, beat the eggs and then mix in the almond milk, honey (or maple syrup), and vanilla extract. Combine the wet and dry ingredients until the batter is smooth.

2. Heat a non-stick skillet or griddle over medium heat and lightly grease with coconut oil or butter. Pour about 1/4 cup of batter

for each pancake. Cook for 2-3 minutes on one side, until bubbles form on the surface, then flip and cook for another 1-2 minutes on the other side. Repeat with remaining batter.

3. Berry Compote: While pancakes are cooking, combine the mixed berries, honey (or maple syrup), and lemon juice in a small saucepan over medium heat. Cook, stirring occasionally, until the berries have softened and the sauce has thickened slightly, about 5-7 minutes.

4. Serve the warm pancakes with the berry compote spooned over the top.

Nutritional Value (per serving, serves 4):

- Calories: Approximately 300 kcal
- Protein: 8g
- Fat: 12g (healthy fats from eggs and coconut flour)
- Carbohydrates: 40g
- Fiber: 10g
- These pancakes are high in fiber and protein, making them a filling and nutritious option for breakfast. The berry compote adds antioxidants and vitamins without the need for processed sugars.

Cooking Time:

- Preparation time: 10 minutes
- Cook time: 15 minutes
- Total time: 25 minutes

Rating: ★★★★★

Coconut Flour Pancakes with Berry Compote offer a delightful twist on traditional pancakes, providing a gluten-free and nutrient-rich start to your day. This dish combines the subtly sweet and fluffy texture of coconut flour pancakes with the tangy freshness of berry compote, creating a breakfast that is as nutritious as it is delicious. Perfect for anyone seeking a healthy, satisfying meal that's quick to prepare, this recipe proves that you can enjoy a gourmet breakfast experience in the comfort of your home, without spending hours in the kitchen.

Baked Apples with Cinnamon and Nuts

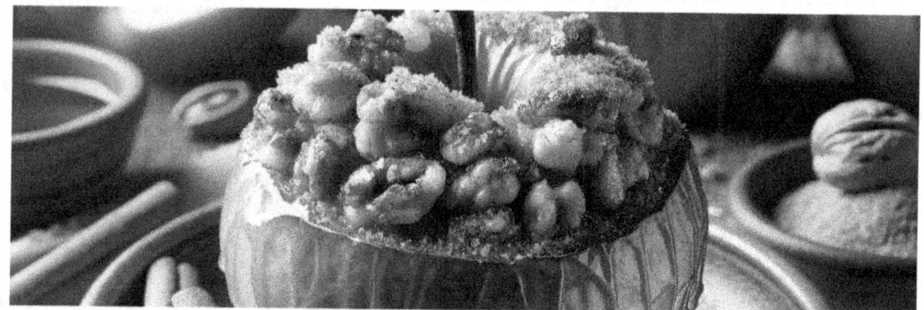

Ingredients:

- 4 large apples, such as Fuji or Gala
- 1/4 cup chopped walnuts or pecans

- 2 tablespoons raisins or dried cranberries (optional)
- 2 tablespoons honey or maple syrup

- 1/2 teaspoon ground cinnamon
- 1/4 teaspoon ground nutmeg
- 1/2 cup water
- Optional toppings: Greek yogurt or whipped cream

Preparation:

1. Core the apples, leaving the bottom intact to create a well. Make a shallow cut around the top of each apple to prevent them from splitting.
2. In a small bowl, mix the chopped nuts, raisins (if using), honey, cinnamon, and nutmeg. Stuff this mixture into the wells of each apple.
3. Place the apples in a deep microwave-safe dish. Pour water into the bottom of the dish to help steam the apples.
4. Microwave on high for 5-6 minutes or until the apples are tender. The exact time may vary depending on your microwave and the size of the apples.
5. Carefully remove the dish from the microwave (it will be hot) and allow the apples to cool slightly.

Nutritional Value (per serving, serves 4):

- Calories: Approximately 180 kcal
- Protein: 1g
- Fat: 4g (healthy fats from nuts)
- Carbohydrates: 38g
- Fiber: 5g

- The nuts add healthy fats and a bit of protein, making this dessert not only delicious but also **nutritious.**

Cooking Time:

- Preparation time: 5 minutes
- Cook time: 6 minutes
- Total time: 11 minutes

Rating: ★★★★★

This quick and healthy version of Baked Apples is perfect for a cozy dessert or a sweet snack. It offers the warm flavors of cinnamon and nutmeg paired with the crunch of nuts and the natural sweetness of apples, all in a fraction of the time it takes to bake them in the oven.

Quick Mango and Chia Seed Pudding

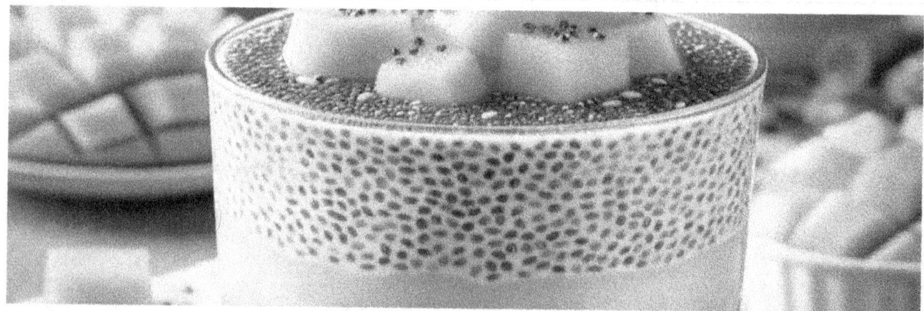

Ingredients:

- 1 ripe mango, peeled and cubed
- 1 cup almond milk (or any plant-based milk of your choice)

- 1/4 cup chia seeds
- 2 tablespoons honey or maple syrup (adjust to taste)
- 1/2 teaspoon vanilla extract
- Optional for garnish: additional mango cubes, coconut flakes, or a sprinkle of cinnamon

Preparation:

1. Reserve a few mango cubes for garnish if desired. Blend the rest of the mango cubes with almond milk, honey (or maple syrup), and vanilla extract until smooth.
2. Pour the mango mixture into a bowl. Stir in chia seeds until well combined.
3. Let the mixture sit for about 5 minutes, then stir again to prevent the chia seeds from clumping.
4. Cover the bowl and refrigerate for at least 20 minutes, or until the pudding has thickened. If you're in a hurry, you can place it in the freezer for about 10-15 minutes, but keep an eye on it to prevent freezing.
5. Serve the pudding in bowls or glasses, garnished with reserved mango cubes, coconut flakes, or a sprinkle of cinnamon, if using.

Nutritional Value (per serving, serves 2):

- Calories: Approximately 250 kcal
- Protein: 5g

- Fat: 7g (healthy fats from chia seeds)
- Carbohydrates: 45g
- Fiber: 10g
- This pudding is rich in omega-3 fatty acids, fiber, and antioxidants, making it a nutritious and satisfying snack or dessert.

Cooking Time:

- Preparation time: 10 minutes
- Chill time: 20 minutes
- Total time: 30 minutes

Rating: ★★★★★

Quick Mango and Chia Seed Pudding is a delightful and nutritious treat that combines the tropical sweetness of mango with the health benefits of chia seeds. This pudding is incredibly easy to make and can be prepared in advance for a convenient breakfast, snack, or dessert. It's a versatile recipe that allows for various toppings, so you can customize it to your liking. Enjoy the creamy texture and sweet flavor of this pudding while benefiting from its wholesome ingredients.

Honey Roasted Pears with Yogurt

Ingredients:

- 4 ripe pears, halved and cored
- 2 tablespoons honey, plus extra for drizzling

- 1/2 teaspoon ground cinnamon
- 1/4 teaspoon ground nutmeg
- 1 cup Greek yogurt for serving
- Optional garnishes: chopped nuts (such as walnuts or almonds), a sprinkle of cinnamon, or fresh berries

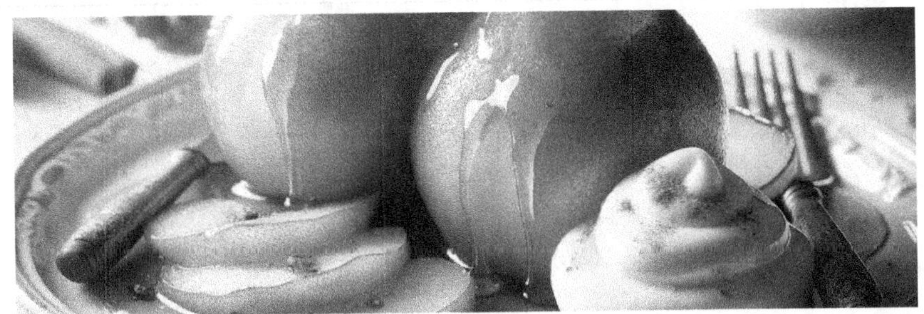

Preparation:

1. Preheat your oven to 375°F (190°C). Line a baking sheet with parchment paper.
2. Place the pear halves cut-side up on the prepared baking sheet.
3. In a small bowl, mix together the honey, cinnamon, and nutmeg. Brush this mixture over the pears, ensuring each half is well coated.
4. Roast in the preheated oven for about 20-25 minutes, or until the pears are tender and caramelized.
5. Serve the roasted pears warm with a dollop of Greek yogurt on the side or on top of each pear half. Drizzle with a little more

honey and add any optional garnishes like chopped nuts, a sprinkle of cinnamon, or fresh berries.

Nutritional Value (per serving, serves 4):

- Calories: Approximately 150 kcal
- Protein: 4g
- Fat: 0.5g
- Carbohydrates: 34g
- Fiber: 5g
- This dessert provides a good source of fiber from the pears and protein from the Greek yogurt, with natural sweetness from the honey.

Cooking Time:

- Preparation time: 5 minutes
- Cook time: 25 minutes
- Total time: 30 minutes

Rating: ★★★★★

Honey Roasted Pears with Yogurt is an elegantly simple and delicious dessert that combines the natural sweetness of pears with the creamy tanginess of Greek yogurt. It's a perfect way to end a meal on a sweet note without overindulgence.

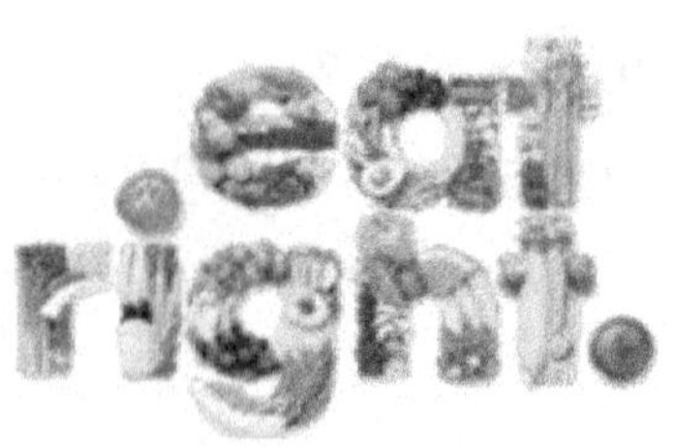

Chapter 8: Soups

In this chapter, we explore a collection of comforting and nourishing soup recipes that are perfect for anyone looking to incorporate healthy, warming dishes into their diet, especially those managing fibromyalgia. Each soup is designed to be prepared in 30 minutes or less, offering a quick and satisfying meal option that doesn't compromise on taste or nutritional value. From the soothing simplicity of a classic vegetable broth to the robust flavors of a spiced pumpkin soup, these recipes are crafted with ingredients known for their anti-inflammatory properties and health benefits. Whether you're seeking a light starter or a hearty main, these soups promise to deliver both comfort and nourishment in every spoonful, making them an ideal choice for any day of the week.

Carrot Ginger Soup

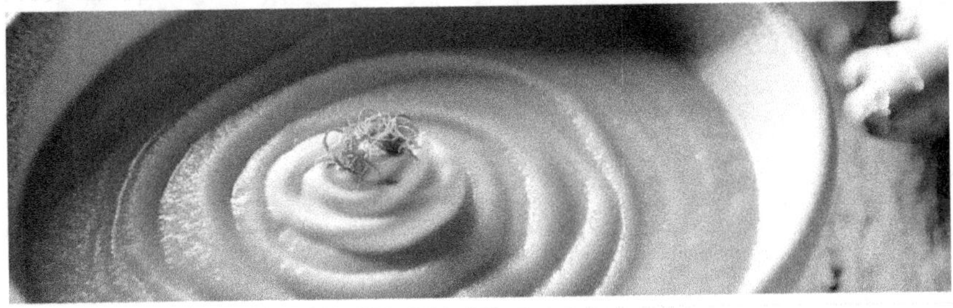

Ingredients:

- 1 tablespoon olive oil
- 1 onion, chopped
- 2 cloves garlic, minced
- 2 tablespoons fresh ginger, grated
- 1-pound carrots, peeled and chopped
- 4 cups vegetable broth
- Salt and pepper to taste
- Optional garnish: fresh parsley or cilantro, a dollop of yogurt or coconut cream

Preparation:

1. Heat the olive oil in a large pot over medium heat. Add the chopped onion and sauté until translucent, about 5 minutes.
2. Add the minced garlic and grated ginger, cooking for another 2 minutes until fragrant.
3. Add the chopped carrots to the pot, stirring to combine with the onion, garlic, and ginger. Cook for 5 minutes, letting the carrots start to soften.
4. Pour in the vegetable broth, and season with salt and pepper. Bring the mixture to a boil, then reduce heat and simmer for 15 minutes, or until the carrots are completely tender.
5. Use an immersion blender to purée the soup directly in the pot, or carefully transfer the mixture to a blender and purée until smooth.

6. Taste and adjust seasoning as needed. Serve hot, garnished with fresh parsley or cilantro and a dollop of yogurt or coconut cream if desired.

Nutritional Value (per serving, serves 4):

- Calories: Approximately 120 kcal
- Protein: 2g
- Fat: 4g (healthy fats from olive oil)
- Carbohydrates: 20g
- Fiber: 5g
- This soup is rich in vitamin A from the carrots and provides anti-inflammatory benefits from the ginger, making it not only delicious but also nutritious.

Cooking Time:

- Preparation time: 10 minutes
- Cook time: 20 minutes
- Total time: 30 minutes

Rating: ★★★★★

Carrot Ginger Soup is a vibrant, flavorful dish that's perfect for a quick and healthy meal. Its soothing qualities and burst of flavors from fresh ginger make it an ideal choice for anyone looking to nourish their body while enjoying a delicious, comforting soup. Easy to make and packed with nutrients, this soup is a wonderful addition to any meal, especially for those managing dietary needs like fibromyalgia.

Tomato and Basil Soup

Ingredients:

- 2 tablespoons olive oil
- 1 onion, diced
- 2 cloves garlic, minced
- 1 can (28 oz) crushed tomatoes
- 2 cups vegetable broth
- 1/4 cup fresh basil leaves, chopped, plus more for garnish
- Salt and pepper to taste
- Optional: 1 teaspoon sugar (to balance acidity)
- Optional for serving: a drizzle of cream or a sprinkle of grated Parmesan cheese

Preparation:

1. Heat the olive oil in a large pot over medium heat. Add the diced onion and sauté until translucent, about 5 minutes.

2. Add the minced garlic and cook for another minute until fragrant.

3. Stir in the crushed tomatoes, vegetable broth, and chopped basil. Season with salt, pepper, and optional sugar to taste. Bring the soup to a simmer.

4. Let the soup simmer for about 15-20 minutes to allow the flavors to meld together.

5. Use an immersion blender to puree the soup directly in the pot to your desired consistency. Alternatively, you can carefully transfer the soup to a blender and puree it in batches.

6. Taste and adjust the seasoning as needed.

7. Serve hot, garnished with fresh basil leaves and optional cream or grated Parmesan cheese.

Nutritional Value (per serving, serves 4):

- Calories: Approximately 150 kcal
- Protein: 3g
- Fat: 7g (healthy fats from olive oil)
- Carbohydrates: 20g
- Fiber: 5g
- This soup is a good source of vitamins A and C from the tomatoes and provides antioxidants from the basil.

Cooking Time:

- Preparation time: 5 minutes
- Carbohydrates: 20g
- Cook time: 25 minutes
- Total time: 30 minutes

Rating: ★★★★★

Tomato and Basil Soup is a classic, comforting dish that's perfect for any season. This quick and easy recipe delivers a rich, flavorful soup that combines the tanginess of tomatoes with the aromatic freshness of basil. Suitable for a light lunch or as a starter for dinner, it's a nutritious option that can be prepared in 30 minutes or less, making it ideal for busy days. Enjoy this heartwarming soup on its own or paired with a crusty piece of bread for a satisfying meal.

Chicken Zoodle Soup

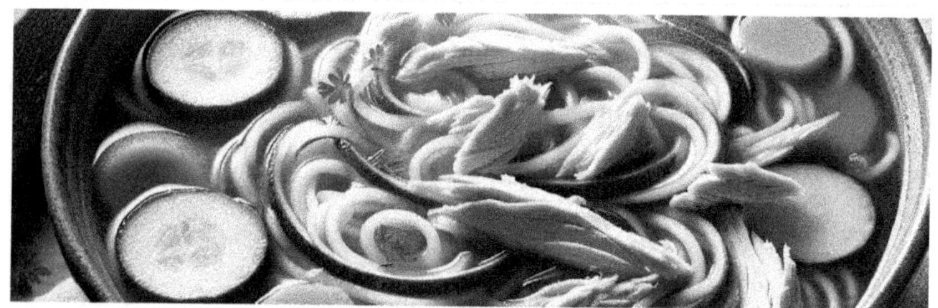

Ingredients:

- 1 tablespoon olive oil
- 1 small onion, diced
- 2 cloves garlic, minced
- 2 medium carrots, peeled and diced
- 2 stalks celery, diced
- 1/2-pound chicken breast, cut into small pieces
- 4 cups chicken broth
- Salt and pepper to taste
- 2 medium zucchinis, spiralized into noodles (zoodles)
- Fresh parsley, chopped, for garnish

Preparation:

1. Heat olive oil in a large pot over medium heat. Add the diced onion, garlic, carrots, and celery. Sauté for about 5 minutes, or until the vegetables are softened.
2. Add the chicken pieces to the pot, seasoning with salt and pepper. Cook until the chicken is no longer pink on the outside, about 5 minutes.
3. Pour in the chicken broth and bring the mixture to a simmer. Let it cook for about 10 minutes, or until the chicken is fully cooked and the vegetables are tender.
4. Add the spiralized zucchini noodles (zoodles) to the pot, and simmer for an additional 2-3 minutes, or just until the zoodles are tender but still firm.
5. Adjust the seasoning with more salt and pepper if needed.
6. Serve the soup hot, garnished with fresh parsley.

Nutritional Value (per serving, serves 4):

- Calories: Approximately 150 kcal
- Protein: 16g
- Fat: 5g (healthy fats from olive oil)
- Carbohydrates: 10g
- Fiber: 2g
- This soup is a light, nutritious option that provides a good source of protein from chicken and a variety of vitamins and minerals from the vegetables.

Cooking Time:

- Preparation time: 5 minutes
- Cook time: 20 minutes
- Total time: 25 minutes

Rating: ★★★★★

Chicken Zoodle Soup is a modern twist on the classic chicken noodle soup, using zucchini noodles for a healthier, low-carb alternative. This soup combines the comforting flavors of traditional chicken soup with the added freshness and nutrition of zoodles, making it an excellent choice for a quick, healthy meal. Perfect for those seeking a satisfying yet light dish, especially suitable for managing dietary needs like fibromyalgia.

Spicy Pumpkin Soup

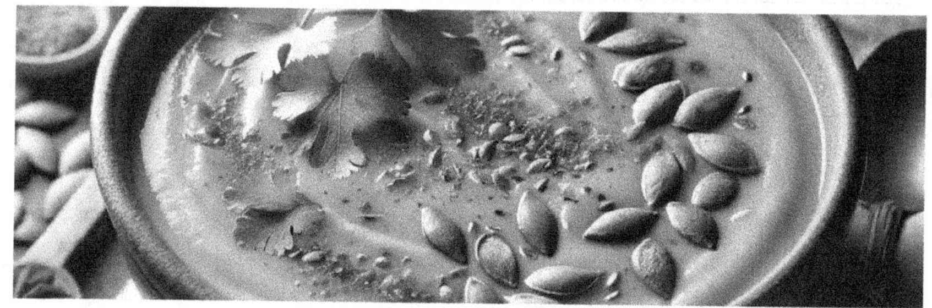

Ingredients:

- 1 tablespoon olive oil
- 1 onion, chopped
- 2 cloves garlic, minced
- 1 teaspoon grated ginger
- 1 teaspoon ground cumin
- 1/2 teaspoon ground coriander
- 1/4 teaspoon cayenne pepper (adjust to taste)

- 1 can (15 oz) pumpkin puree (not pumpkin pie filling)
- 4 cups vegetable broth
- Salt and pepper to taste
- 1 can (14 oz) coconut milk
- Optional garnishes: roasted pumpkin seeds, fresh cilantro, or a swirl of coconut milk

Preparation:

1. Heat the olive oil in a large pot over medium heat. Add the chopped onion and sauté until translucent, about 5 minutes.
2. Add the minced garlic, grated ginger, cumin, coriander, and cayenne pepper. Cook for another 2 minutes, stirring frequently, until fragrant.
3. Stir in the pumpkin puree and vegetable broth. Season with salt and pepper. Bring the mixture to a simmer.
4. Let the soup simmer for about 15 minutes to meld the flavors together.
5. Stir in the coconut milk, reserving a little for garnish if desired, and heat through without boiling.
6. Use an immersion blender to puree the soup until smooth, or carefully transfer to a blender in batches.
7. Taste and adjust seasoning as needed. Serve hot, garnished with roasted pumpkin seeds, fresh cilantro, or a swirl of coconut milk.

Nutritional Value (per serving, serves 4):

- Calories: Approximately 250 kcal
- Protein: 3g
- Fat: 18g (healthy fats from olive oil and coconut milk)
- Carbohydrates: 20g

- Fiber: 5g
- This soup is a good source of vitamins A and C, fiber, and healthy fats, making it both nourishing and comforting.

Cooking Time:

- Preparation time: 5 minutes

- Cook time: 20 minutes
- Total time: 25 minutes

Rating: ★★★★★

Spicy Pumpkin Soup is a creamy, flavorful dish that brings warmth and comfort with every spoonful. Infused with exotic spices and enriched with coconut milk, this soup offers a delightful balance of sweet and spicy flavors. Easy to prepare in under 30 minutes, it's an ideal choice for a quick, satisfying meal, especially on chilly days. Whether you're seeking a cozy dinner option or a festive autumnal dish, this spicy pumpkin soup is sure to please.

Broccoli and Pea Soup with Mint

Ingredients:

- 1 tablespoon olive oil
- 1 onion, chopped

- 2 cloves garlic, minced
- 3 cups broccoli florets

- 1 cup frozen peas
- 4 cups vegetable broth
- Salt and pepper to taste
- 1/4 cup fresh mint leaves, plus extra for garnish
- Optional: Greek yogurt or a swirl of cream for serving

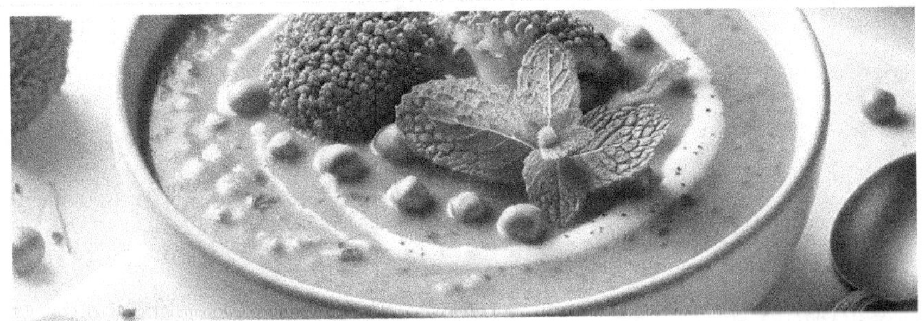

Preparation:

1. Heat the olive oil in a large pot over medium heat. Add the chopped onion and sauté until translucent, about 5 minutes.

2. Add the minced garlic and cook for another minute until fragrant.

3. Add the broccoli florets, frozen peas, and vegetable broth to the pot. Season with salt and pepper. Bring to a boil, then reduce heat and simmer for about 10 minutes, or until the broccoli is tender.

4. Stir in the fresh mint leaves.

5. Use an immersion blender to puree the soup directly in the pot until smooth. Alternatively, carefully transfer the soup to a blender and puree in batches.

6. Taste and adjust the seasoning as needed.

7. Serve hot, garnished with additional mint leaves and a dollop of Greek yogurt or a swirl of cream if desired.

Nutritional Value (per serving, serves 4):

- Calories: Approximately 120 kcal

- Protein: 5g

- Fat: 4g (healthy fats from olive oil)

- Carbohydrates: 17g

- Fiber: 5g

- This soup is rich in vitamins C and K, fiber, and antioxidants, making it a healthy and refreshing choice.

Cooking Time:

- Preparation time: 5 minutes

- Cook time: 15 minutes

- **Total time: 20 minutes**

Rating: ★★★★★

Broccoli and Pea Soup with Mint is a vibrant, flavorful dish perfect for a light lunch or a healthy start to any meal. Its bright green color and refreshing taste make it a delightful option for those seeking nutritious and quick recipes.

Chapter 9: Salads

Welcome to the Salads chapter, a vibrant collection of dishes that celebrate the freshness and diversity of ingredients that can support and nourish the body, especially for those navigating the challenges of fibromyalgia. Understanding the importance of anti-inflammatory foods and nutrients in managing symptoms, we've curated a selection of salads that are not only quick to assemble—ready in 30 minutes or less—but also packed with flavors and textures to delight your taste buds. From leafy greens adorned with colorful vegetables and lean proteins to grains and legumes enhanced with herbs and spices, each recipe is designed to offer a balanced meal or side that's both satisfying and healthful. Dive into these pages to discover how salads can be a cornerstone of a diet that fosters well-being and vitality, proving that quick, nutritious meals can also be incredibly delicious.

Spinach and Strawberry Salad with Walnuts

Ingredients:

- 4 cups fresh spinach leaves, washed and dried
- 1 cup strawberries, hulled and sliced
- 1/4 cup walnuts, chopped
- 2 tablespoons balsamic vinegar
- 1 tablespoon extra-virgin olive oil
- 1 teaspoon honey or maple syrup
- Salt and pepper to taste

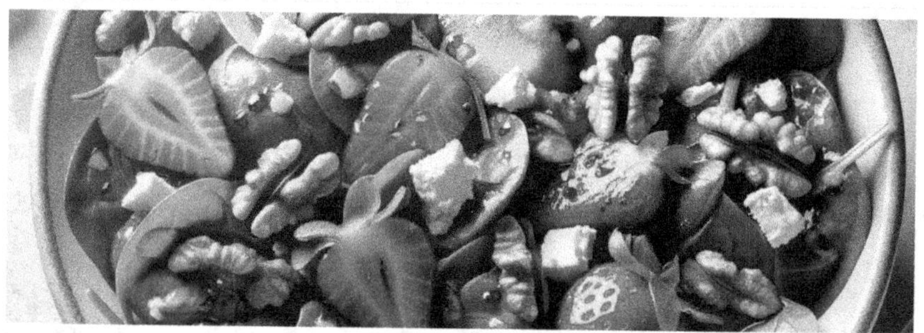

Preparation:

1. In a large salad bowl, combine the fresh spinach leaves, sliced strawberries, and chopped walnuts.

2. In a small bowl, whisk together the balsamic vinegar, extra virgin olive oil, honey or maple syrup, salt, and pepper to make the dressing.

3. Drizzle the dressing over the salad ingredients and toss gently to coat evenly.

4. Serve immediately, garnished with additional walnuts if desired.

Nutritional Value (per serving, serves 2):

- Calories: Approximately 200 kcal
- Protein: 4g
- Fat: 15g (healthy fats from walnuts and olive oil)
- Carbohydrates: 15g
- Fiber: 4g

Preparation Time: 10 minutes

Rating: ★★★★★

- This salad is rich in vitamins, minerals, antioxidants, and healthy fats, providing a refreshing and nourishing meal option.

Spinach and Strawberry Salad with Walnuts is a delightful combination of flavors and textures that's perfect for a quick and nutritious meal. The sweetness of the strawberries complements the earthiness of the spinach, while the crunch of the walnuts adds a satisfying contrast.

Mediterranean Quinoa Salad

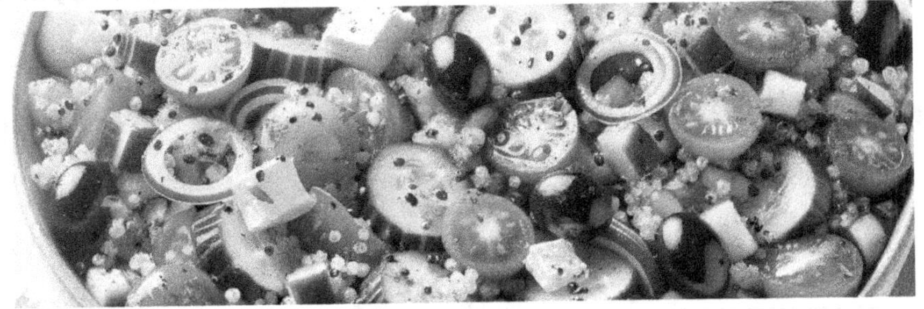

Ingredients:

- 1 cup quinoa, rinsed

- 2 cups water or vegetable broth
- 1 cup cherry tomatoes, halved
- 1 cucumber, diced
- 1/2 cup Kalamata olives, pitted and sliced
- 1/4 cup red onion, finely chopped
- 1/4 cup fresh parsley, chopped
- 1/4 cup feta cheese, crumbled
- Juice of 1 lemon
- 2 tablespoons extra virgin olive oil
- 1 clove garlic, minced
- 1 teaspoon dried oregano
- Salt and pepper to taste

Preparation:

1. In a medium saucepan, bring the water or vegetable broth to a boil. Add the quinoa, reduce heat to low, cover, and simmer for 15-20 minutes, or until the quinoa is cooked and the liquid is absorbed. Remove from heat and let it cool.

2. In a large salad bowl, combine the cooked quinoa, cherry tomatoes, cucumber, Kalamata olives, red onion, and parsley.

3. In a small bowl, whisk together the lemon juice, extra virgin olive oil, minced garlic, dried oregano, salt, and pepper to make the dressing.

4. Pour the dressing over the salad ingredients and toss gently to coat evenly.

5. Sprinkle the crumbled feta cheese over the top of the salad before serving.

Nutritional Value (per serving, serves 4):

- Calories: Approximately 250 kcal
- Protein: 8g
- Fat: 10g (healthy fats from olive oil and feta cheese)
- Carbohydrates: 30g
- Fiber: 5g
- This salad is rich in protein, fiber, vitamins, and minerals, providing a satisfying and nutritious meal option.

Preparation Time: 20 minutes

Rating: ★★★★★

Mediterranean Quinoa Salad is a colorful and flavorful dish that's bursting with the vibrant tastes of the Mediterranean. Packed with protein-rich quinoa, crisp vegetables, tangy olives, and creamy feta cheese, this salad offers a satisfying and nutritious meal that's perfect for lunch or dinner. The zesty dressing, made with lemon juice, garlic, and olive oil, adds a refreshing burst of flavor that ties everything together beautifully. Whether you're a fan of Mediterranean cuisine or simply looking for a healthy and delicious salad option, this recipe is sure to impress.

Beetroot and Goat Cheese Salad

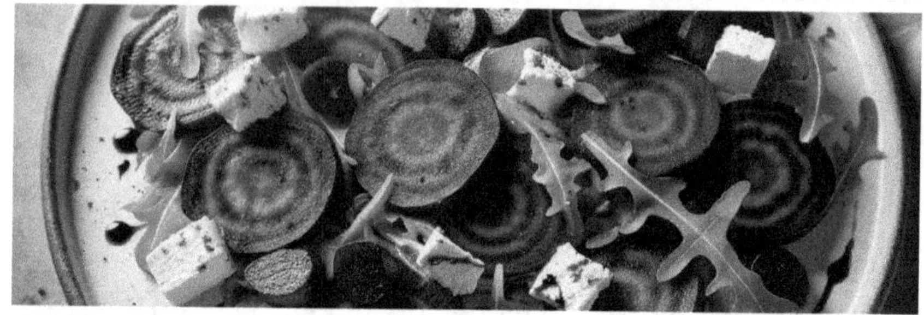

Ingredients:

- 2 medium beetroots, cooked and sliced
- 4 cups mixed salad greens (such as arugula, spinach, or mixed baby greens)
- 1/4 cup walnuts, chopped
- 2 ounces goat cheese, crumbled
- 2 tablespoons balsamic vinegar
- 2 tablespoons extra virgin olive oil
- 1 teaspoon honey or maple syrup
- Salt and pepper to taste

Preparation:

1. If the beetroots are not already cooked, wrap them individually in aluminum foil and roast in a preheated oven at 400°F (200°C) for about 45-60 minutes, or until tender when pierced with a fork. Let them cool, then peel and slice them.

2. In a large salad bowl, combine the mixed salad greens, sliced beetroots, and chopped walnuts.

3. In a small bowl, whisk together the balsamic vinegar, extra virgin olive oil, honey or maple syrup, salt, and pepper to make the dressing.
4. Drizzle the dressing over the salad ingredients and toss gently to coat evenly.
5. Sprinkle the crumbled goat cheese over the top of the salad before serving.

Nutritional Value (per serving, serves 2):

- Calories: Approximately 300 kcal
- Protein: 8g
- Fat: 22g (healthy fats from walnuts and olive oil)
- Carbohydrates: 20g
- Fiber: 6g
- This salad is rich in vitamins, minerals, antioxidants, and healthy fats, providing a delicious and nutritious meal option.

Preparation Time: 15 minutes (if beetroots are pre-cooked)

Rating: ★★★★★

Beetroot and Goat Cheese Salad is a vibrant and flavorful dish that's both visually stunning and delicious. The earthy sweetness of the beetroot pairs beautifully with the creamy tanginess of the goat cheese, while the crunchy walnuts add texture and depth. Tossed with a simple balsamic vinaigrette, this salad is a perfect balance of flavors and textures. Whether served as a light lunch or a refreshing side dish, it's sure to impress with its vibrant colors and delicious taste.

Kale, Avocado, and Quinoa Salad

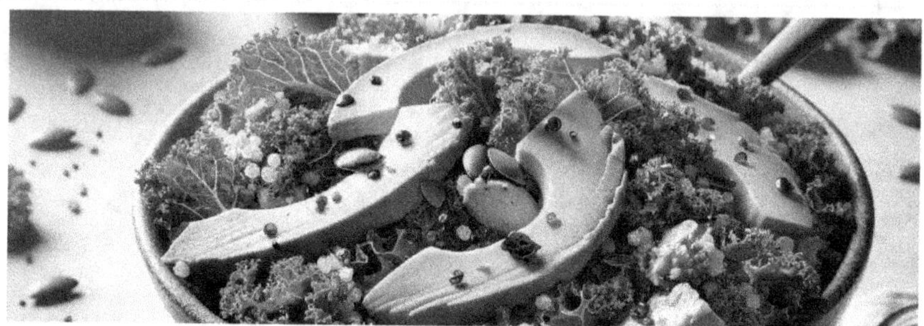

Ingredients:

- 1 cup quinoa, rinsed
- 2 cups water or vegetable broth
- 4 cups kale leaves, stems removed and chopped
- 1 avocado, diced
- 1/4 cup dried cranberries
- 1/4 cup sliced almonds
- Juice of 1 lemon
- 2 tablespoons extra virgin olive oil
- 1 clove garlic, minced
- Salt and pepper to taste

Preparation:

1. In a medium saucepan, bring the water or vegetable broth to a boil. Add the quinoa, reduce heat to low, cover, and simmer for 15-20 minutes, or until the quinoa is cooked and the liquid is absorbed. Remove from heat and let it cool.

2. In a large salad bowl, combine the chopped kale leaves, diced avocado, dried cranberries, and sliced almonds.

3. In a small bowl, whisk together the lemon juice, extra virgin olive oil, minced garlic, salt, and pepper to make the dressing.

4. Pour the dressing over the salad ingredients and toss gently to coat evenly.

5. Add the cooked quinoa to the salad and toss again to combine.

6. Serve immediately, or refrigerate for later.

Nutritional Value (per serving, serves 4):

- Calories: Approximately 300 kcal
- Protein: 8g
- Fat: 15g (healthy fats from avocado, olive oil, and almonds)
- Carbohydrates: 35g
- Fiber: 8g
- This salad is rich in protein, fiber, vitamins, and minerals, providing a satisfying and nutritious meal option.

Preparation Time: 20 minutes

Rating: ★★★★★

Kale, Avocado, and Quinoa Salad is a nutrient-packed dish that's both delicious and satisfying. The combination of hearty kale, creamy avocado, protein-rich quinoa, and crunchy almonds creates a flavorful and texturally diverse salad that's sure to please your taste buds. Dressed with a zesty lemon garlic vinaigrette and dotted with sweet dried cranberries, this salad is a perfect balance of flavors and textures. Whether enjoyed as a light lunch or a hearty side dish, it's a versatile recipe that's quick and easy to prepare, making it an excellent choice for busy days.

Cucumber Noodle Prawn Salad

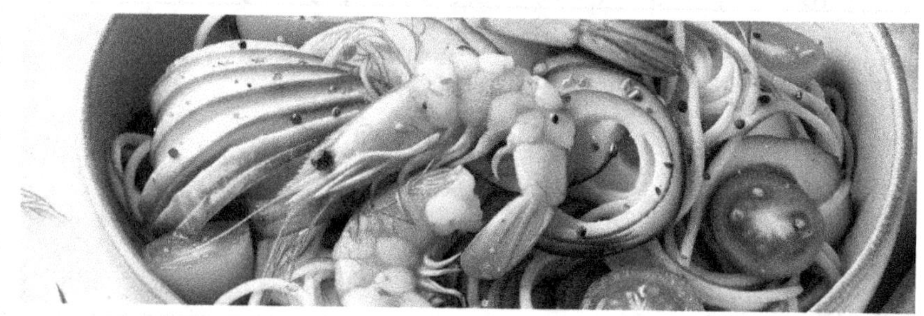

Ingredients:

- 1 large cucumber, spiralized into noodles
- 8 ounces cooked prawns (shrimp), peeled and deveined
- 1 red bell pepper, thinly sliced
- 1/4 cup fresh cilantro leaves, chopped
- 1/4 cup chopped peanuts or cashews
- 2 tablespoons sesame seeds (optional, for garnish)

For the dressing:

- 2 tablespoons soy sauce (or tamari for gluten-free option)
- 1 tablespoon rice vinegar
- 1 tablespoon honey or maple syrup
- 1 tablespoon sesame oil
- 1 clove garlic, minced
- 1 teaspoon grated ginger
- 1 teaspoon sriracha sauce (adjust to taste)

Preparation:

1. In a large bowl, combine the cucumber noodles, cooked prawns, sliced red bell pepper, and chopped cilantro.
2. In a small bowl, whisk together the soy sauce, rice vinegar, honey or maple syrup, sesame oil, minced garlic, grated ginger, and sriracha sauce to make the dressing.
3. Pour the dressing over the salad ingredients and toss gently to coat evenly.
4. Sprinkle chopped peanuts or cashews over the salad before serving.
5. Optionally, garnish with sesame seeds for added texture and flavor.

Nutritional Value (per serving, serves 2):

- Calories: Approximately 300 kcal
- Protein: 25g
- Fat: 15g (healthy fats from nuts and sesame oil)
- Carbohydrates: 20g
- Fiber: 5g

- This salad is rich in protein, healthy fats, and vitamins, providing a satisfying and nutritious meal option.

Preparation Time: 15 minutes

Rating: ★★★★★

Cucumber Noodle Prawn Salad is a refreshing and light dish that's perfect for a quick and satisfying meal. The combination of crisp cucumber noodles, succulent prawns, crunchy bell peppers, and aromatic cilantro creates a burst of flavors and textures in every bite. Tossed with a tangy and spicy dressing, this salad is both delicious and nutritious. Whether served as a main course or a side dish, it's sure to impress with its vibrant colors and delightful taste. Plus, it's quick and easy to prepare, making it an excellent choice for busy weeknights or lunch on the go

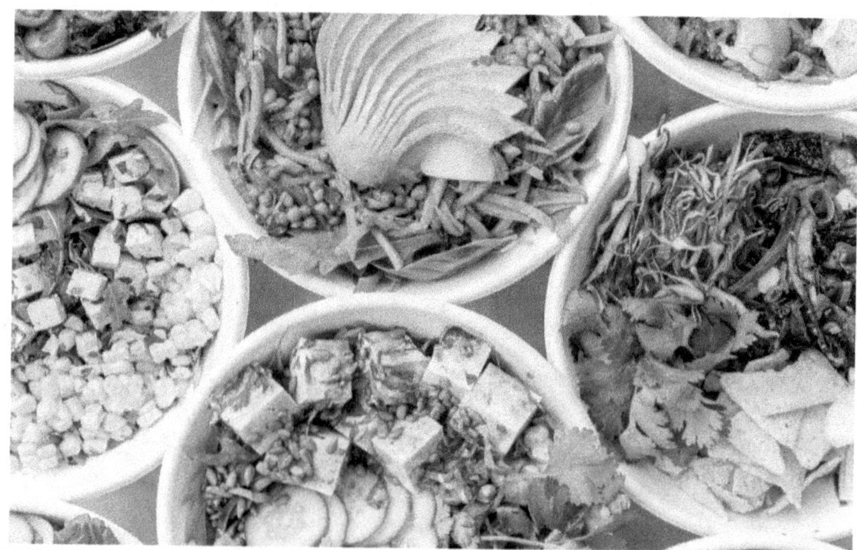

Chapter 10: Implementing a Fibromyalgia-Friendly Diet

Adopting a fibromyalgia-specific diet entails learning your body's sensitivities to various foods and focusing on options that relieve pain. This simple guide can help you navigate your dietary changes for improved symptom management.

Listen to your body. Begin by determining which foods exacerbate or alleviate your symptoms. A food journal can be an effective tool in the discovery process.

Anti-Inflammatory Foods: Include foods high in omega-3 fatty acids, antioxidants, and fiber, such as fatty fish, fresh fruits and vegetables, and whole grains. These can assist in relieving inflammation and discomfort.

Reduce Inflammatory meals: Avoid processed meals, refined carbohydrates, and saturated fats, which can worsen fibromyalgia symptoms.

Stay Hydrated: Drinking lots of water is critical for controlling fibromyalgia, as it aids digestion and general well-being.

Meal Planning and Cooking: Plan your meals with fibromyalgia-friendly foods. Batch cooking and basic preparation techniques can save time and energy.

To treat any nutritional deficiencies, contact a healthcare expert before taking supplements such as Vitamin D and magnesium.

Be Patient and Seek Support: Making dietary adjustments takes time. Seek help from healthcare experts or support organizations to make the transition easier.

Implementing these dietary guidelines can greatly improve your fibromyalgia management, resulting in fewer symptoms and a higher quality of life.

7 Days Sample Meal Plan

Day 1:

Breakfast: Overnight Oats with Berries and Chia Seeds

Lunch: Turmeric Chicken Salad Wrap

Dinner: Garlic Ginger Shrimp Stir-Fry

Snack: Almond and Flaxseed Energy Balls

Day 2:

Breakfast: Avocado Toast with Poached Eggs

Lunch: Quick Lentil and Vegetable Soup

Dinner: Lemon Herb Baked Cod

Snack: Sweet Potato and Kale Chips

Day 3:

Breakfast: Quinoa Porridge with Almonds and Honey

Lunch: Chickpea and Avocado Salad

Dinner: Chicken and Broccoli Alfredo (Gluten-Free)

Snack: Cucumber and Hummus Bites

Day 4:

Breakfast: Anti-Inflammatory Smoothie Bowls

Lunch: Quinoa and Black Bean Stuffed Peppers

Dinner: Zucchini Noodles with Pesto and Cherry Tomatoes

Snack: Quinoa Tabbouleh

Day 5:

Breakfast: Quick Spinach and Feta Scrambled Eggs

Lunch: Easy Salmon and Avocado Salad

Dinner: Spicy Tofu and Mushroom Bowl

Snack: Baked Zucchini Fries

Day 6:

Breakfast: Coconut Flour Pancakes with Berry Compote

Lunch: Pan-Seared Scallops with Lemon Butter Sauce

Dinner: Quick Chicken Parmesan

Snack: Avocado Chocolate Mousse

Day 7:

Breakfast: Quick Mango and Chia Seed Pudding

Lunch: Tilapia with Mango Salsa

Dinner: Spiced Lamb Chops with Yogurt Sauce

Snack: Honey Roasted Pears with Yogurt

This meal plan offers a variety of flavorful and nutritious meals throughout the week, incorporating a range of ingredients to support overall health and well-being. Enjoy experimenting with these recipes and feel free to adjust based on personal preferences and dietary needs.

Meal Planning and Preparation Tips

Meal planning and preparation are essential for keeping a balanced diet, saving time, and lowering stress at meal times. Here are some methods to simplify your meal planning and preparation process:

Set aside a dedicated day each week to arrange your meals. This covers breakfast, lunch, supper, and snacks. Planning ahead of time helps you avoid making poor decisions at the last minute.

Make a Meal Calendar: Use a computer app or a basic paper calendar to plan your meals for the week. This visual guide can help you buy and prepare more effectively.

Create a Go-To Recipe List: Make a list of your favorite healthy, easy-to-make dishes. Having a recipe repertoire might help you organize your meals more efficiently.

Shop Smart: Create a shopping list based on your meal plan to ensure that you only buy what you need. Stick to the list to prevent making impulsive purchases that may not fit into your healthy eating plan.

Prepare Ingredients in Bulk: After buying, wash, cut, and store veggies and fruits. Cook grains and proteins in bulk. This upfront effort cuts cooking time over the week.

Use Leftovers: Make extra portions of certain dishes so you can consume them for lunch the next day or freeze them for later use.

Embrace Batch Cooking: Prepare full meals in advance and freeze them in parts. This method is especially handy during hectic periods where cooking time is restricted.

Invest in Quality Storage: Keep a variety of containers on hand to store prepared foods and leftovers. Clear containers allow you to see what's within, making it easier to use what you already have.

Keep your cupboard stocked with essentials such as whole grains, canned beans, spices, and healthy oils. These basic ingredients may be used to make a variety of dishes.

Use Technology: There are several applications and online tools available to assist with meal planning and tracking. Look over these resources to see which one works best for you.

Make It a Family Event: If feasible, include family members in meal planning and preparation. This can make the procedure more fun and manageable.

Be Adaptable: Sometimes plans change. Prepare some fast and healthy alternatives on days when cooking is not feasible, such as frozen vegetables, pre-cooked cereals, or canned fish.

By incorporating these meal planning and preparation strategies into your daily routine, you can make healthy eating more doable and pleasurable, even on the busiest days.

Understanding Food Labels and Ingredients to Avoid

Understanding food labels is critical for making educated dietary decisions, especially when attempting to avoid specific substances due to health concerns, allergies, or personal preferences. Here's how to navigate food labels and find substances to avoid:

Read Food Labels

Food labels are separated into two sections: the Nutrition Facts panel, which contains information on calories, fats, carbohydrates, and other important nutrients, and the ingredient list, which lists all of the components in the product by weight, from most to least.

Key Components to Watch:

Serving Size: The quantity considered a single serving. All of the nutritional information on the label is based on this quantity.

Calories: The energy value of one serving. Adjust your consumption according to your dietary needs.

Pay attention to saturated and trans fats, cholesterol, salt, and sweets. These should be limited.

Fiber and Protein: Choose meals strong in fiber and protein since they are more satisfying and provide several health advantages.

Ingredients to Avoid.

Certain substances might impair or worsen health disorders such as fibromyalgia, allergies, and cardiovascular disease. Here are some frequent ones to watch out for:

Trans Fats: Also known as "partially hydrogenated oils," they are strongly connected to heart disease and should be avoided.

High fructose corn syrup (HFCS) is a form of added sugar that has been linked to obesity, diabetes, and other health concerns.

Sodium: High sodium levels can cause hypertension and cardiovascular illness. Aim for goods that contain less than 200 mg of salt per serving.

Artificial Sweeteners: While regulatory bodies deem them safe, some people choose to avoid them owing to potential health risks or sensitivities.

Artificial Colors and Preservatives: Some people are sensitive to these additions and may have negative effects.

Monosodium Glutamate (MSG) is known to induce headaches and allergic reactions in some people.

Gluten: If you have fibromyalgia or are gluten-sensitive avoid goods containing wheat, barley, or rye.

Tips to Avoid Unwanted Ingredients

Prioritize whole foods. Focusing on complete, unadulterated meals reduces your exposure to unnecessary additives.

Learn Synonyms: Some substances can be mentioned under many names. Sugar, for example, can take several forms, including cane syrup, inverted sugar, maltose, and so on.

Check for Allergen Statements: These are often included underneath the ingredient list and indicate common allergies such as nuts, dairy, and soy.

Using Apps: Several mobile apps can scan barcodes and indicate potentially harmful components according to your choices.

Learning to read food labels may help you make better nutritional choices, avoid undesired additives, and manage health issues or dietary restrictions. This information enables you to take charge of your nutrition and make decisions that are consistent with your health goals.

Staying Hydrated and Other Lifestyle Tips

Staying hydrated and practicing certain lifestyle choices may have a significant influence on your overall health and well-being. Here are some important recommendations for staying hydrated and improving your lifestyle.

Staying Hydrated

Understand Your Needs: While the frequently advised eight glasses of water per day is a reasonable beginning point, individual requirements vary depending on factors such as activity level, climate, and health state.

Carry a Water Bottle: Having water on hand motivates you to drink more throughout the day.

Eat Water-Rich Foods. Cucumbers, oranges, strawberries, and lettuce may all help you drink enough water every day.

Monitor Hydration Levels: Pay attention to your body's cues, such as thirst and the color of your urine, which should be pale yellow.

Limit Dehydrating Beverages: Reduce your intake of alcohol, coffee, and sugary drinks, which can all lead to dehydration.

Nutrition

Eat a Balanced Diet: To guarantee a diverse range of necessary nutrients, eat a variety of foods such as whole grains, lean proteins, healthy fats, and lots of fruits and vegetables.

Mind Your Portions: Understanding portion proportions will help you avoid overeating and keep a healthy weight.

Physical activity.

Stay Active: Aim for at least 150 minutes of moderate aerobic activity or 75 minutes of strenuous activity each week, as well as muscle-strengthening activities twice or more per week.

Find Activities You Enjoy: If you love exercising, you are more likely to continue doing so. Try several activities to see what you enjoy most.

Aim for 7-9 hours of quality sleep every night to improve recovery, mood, and cognitive performance.

Establish a Routine: Going to bed and getting up at the same time every day can help regulate your internal clock and enhance your sleep quality.

Stress Management Practice: Mindfulness techniques, such as meditation, deep breathing, and yoga, can help to decrease stress and promote mental health.

Take Pauses: Taking small pauses during the day might help you manage stress and increase productivity.

Social Connections

Maintain Relationships: Strong social relationships are critical for mental wellness. Invest time in developing and sustaining relationships with family and friends.

Seek Help When Needed: When coping with stress or mental health concerns, do not be afraid to seek professional help or the support of loved ones.

Limit screen time.

Be Mindful About Screen Use. Excessive screen usage can disrupt your sleep and mental wellness. Try to restrict your screen usage, especially before bedtime.

Incorporating these hydration and lifestyle guidelines into your daily routine will help you improve your physical health, emotional well-being, and general quality of life. Remember that minor, persistent adjustments can provide huge long-term advantages.

Supplements and Nutrients of Interest for Fibromyalgia

Individuals with fibromyalgia have everyday challenges in managing symptoms such as widespread pain, exhaustion, and sleep difficulties. While there is no one-size-fits-all treatment, several vitamins and minerals have been discovered as possibly helpful in relieving specific fibromyalgia symptoms. However, before beginning any new supplement regimen, talk with a healthcare professional to avoid interactions with medicines or other negative effects.

Magnesium

Magnesium is essential for muscular function, neuronal communication, and improving sleep quality. According to some studies, magnesium coupled with malic acid may help lessen fibromyalgia pain and sensitivity.

Vitamin D

Vitamin D insufficiency is frequent in persons with fibromyalgia, and some research has connected low vitamin D levels to increased pain. Supplementing with vitamin D may alleviate symptoms such as pain and sadness.

Omega 3 Fatty Acids

Fish oil contains omega-3 fatty acids, which have anti-inflammatory qualities and may help reduce fibromyalgia symptoms. They can also aid with mood and cognitive function, which is important for those with fibro fog.

Coenzyme Q-10 (CoQ10)

CoQ10 is an antioxidant that aids energy production in your cells. According to research, CoQ10 supplementation may lessen fibromyalgia sufferers' pain, fatigue, and morning lethargy.

SAMe (S-Adenosylmethionine)

SAMe is a naturally occurring molecule found in the body that has a role in various metabolic processes. It has been investigated for its impact on depression and osteoarthritis, with some data indicating that it may also help alleviate fibromyalgia symptoms.

5-HTP (Hydroxytryptophan)

5-HTP is a precursor of serotonin, a neurotransmitter that controls mood, sleep, and pain. Supplementing with 5-HTP may assist in enhancing sleep quality, mood, and pain tolerance.

Melatonin

Melatonin pills can help fibromyalgia people sleep better. Better sleep can lead to fewer symptoms and a higher quality of life.

Probiotics

Gut health influences overall health and may be especially important in fibromyalgia. Probiotics can help maintain a healthy gut microbiota, which may influence inflammation and immunological function.

Turmeric (curcumin)

Turmeric includes curcumin, which has powerful anti-inflammatory and antioxidant effects. It may help decrease pain and inflammation, but additional study is needed in the case of fibromyalgia.

Tips for Supplementation

Consult a Healthcare Provider. Before adding any supplements to your routine, consult with your healthcare professional to confirm they are appropriate for your needs.

Quality Matters: Select high-quality supplements from reputed suppliers to guarantee safety and efficacy.

Start Slowly: Begin with a modest dose and gradually increase as directed by a healthcare expert to reduce any negative effects.

Monitor your Symptoms: Keep track of any changes in your symptoms or side effects from supplements, and alter your regimen as necessary under the supervision of a healthcare expert.

Incorporating certain vitamins and minerals into your fibromyalgia treatment regimen may provide further relief from symptoms. However, supplements should be used in conjunction with, not instead of, any therapies and lifestyle changes recommended by your healthcare team.

Shopping List for a Fibromyalgia-Friendly Pantry

Creating a fibromyalgia-friendly pantry starts with choosing foods that can help manage symptoms and improve overall well-being. Focus on anti-inflammatory foods, high-quality proteins, whole grains, and a variety of fruits and vegetables. Here's a shopping list to help you stock a kitchen that supports your health journey with fibromyalgia:

Fruits and Vegetables

- Leafy greens (spinach, kale, Swiss chard)
- Berries (strawberries, blueberries, raspberries)
- Cherries
- Oranges
- Apples
- Avocados
- Sweet potatoes
- Broccoli
- Bell peppers

Whole Grains

- Quinoa
- Brown rice
- Oats
- Whole grain pasta

- Barley

Proteins

- Lean chicken or turkey
- Fish rich in omega-3 fatty acids (salmon, mackerel, sardines)
- Legumes (lentils, chickpeas, black beans)
- Eggs
- Tofu or tempeh (for plant-based options)

Healthy Fats

- Extra virgin olive oil
- Coconut oil
- Avocado oil
- Nuts (almonds, walnuts, cashews)
- Seeds (flaxseeds, chia seeds, pumpkin seeds)

Dairy or Dairy Alternatives

- Greek yogurt (opt for plain, and low or full-fat based on your dietary needs)
- Almond milk, soy milk, or oat milk (unsweetened)
- Cheese (in moderation, look for low-lactose options if sensitive)

Herbs, Spices, and Condiments

- Turmeric (curcumin)
- Ginger
- Garlic
- Cinnamon

- Black pepper (to enhance the absorption of turmeric)

- Honey (in moderation)
- Apple cider vinegar

Snacks and Others

- Dark chocolate (at least 70% cocoa)
- Air-popped popcorn

- Rice cakes
- Herbal teas (ginger, peppermint, green tea)

Supplements and Superfoods (Consult with a Healthcare Provider)

- Magnesium
- Omega-3 supplements (fish oil or algae-based for vegetarians)

- Vitamin D
- Probiotic supplements

Beverages

- Plenty of water

- Herbal teas

Foods to Limit or Avoid

- Processed foods and snacks
- High-sugar foods and beverages
- Fried foods

- High-sodium products
- Alcohol
- Caffeine (limit intake if sensitive)

Remember, this list is a guideline. Individual tolerances and dietary needs vary, so it's essential to listen to your body and adjust accordingly. Experimenting with different foods and noting how they affect your symptoms can help you tailor your diet to best support your fibromyalgia management. Always consult with a healthcare provider before making significant dietary changes or adding new supplements to your regimen.

SCAN TO ACCESS MORE AMAZING COOKBOOKS FROM JOAN

For further Questions and advice reach out on
joanmilonehelpdesk@gmail.com

Thank You

I'm writing this with a heart full of gratitude for your kind words and the time you took to read my book, knowing that my words have resonated with you is a reward beyond measure. Thank you again for your appreciation and for being a part of this literary journey.

Warmly,

Joan

30 Days
Meal
Planner

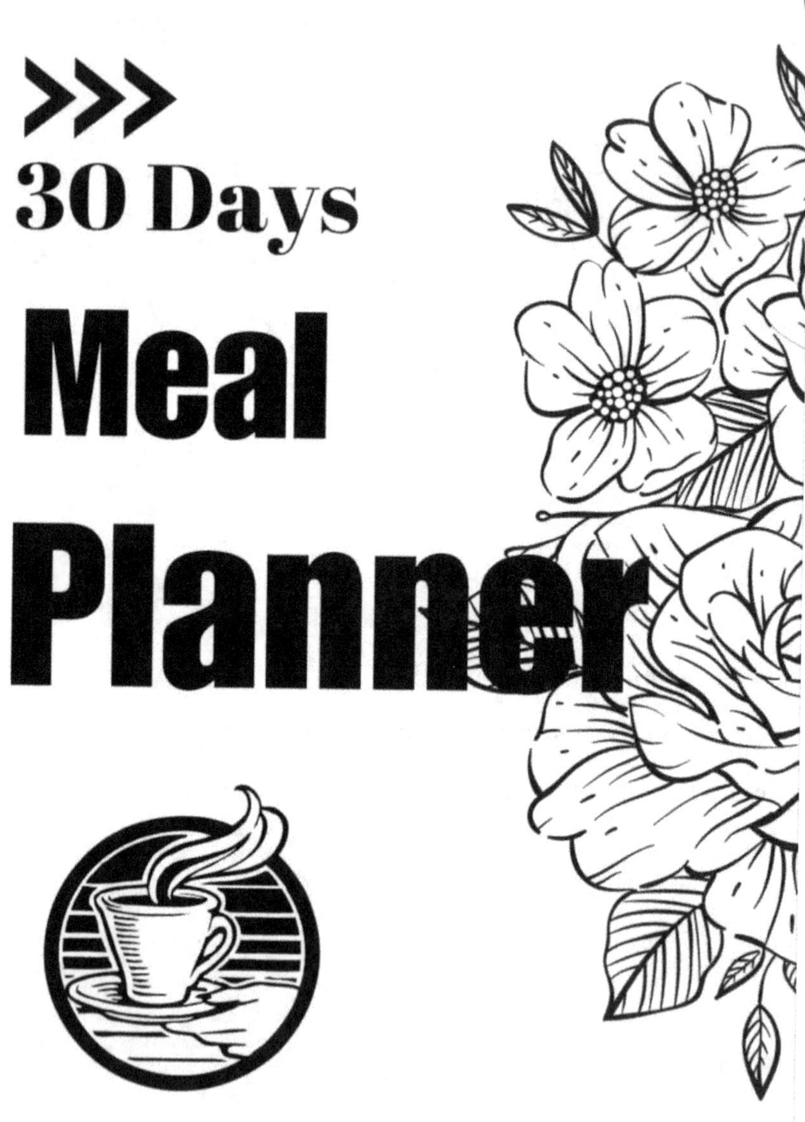

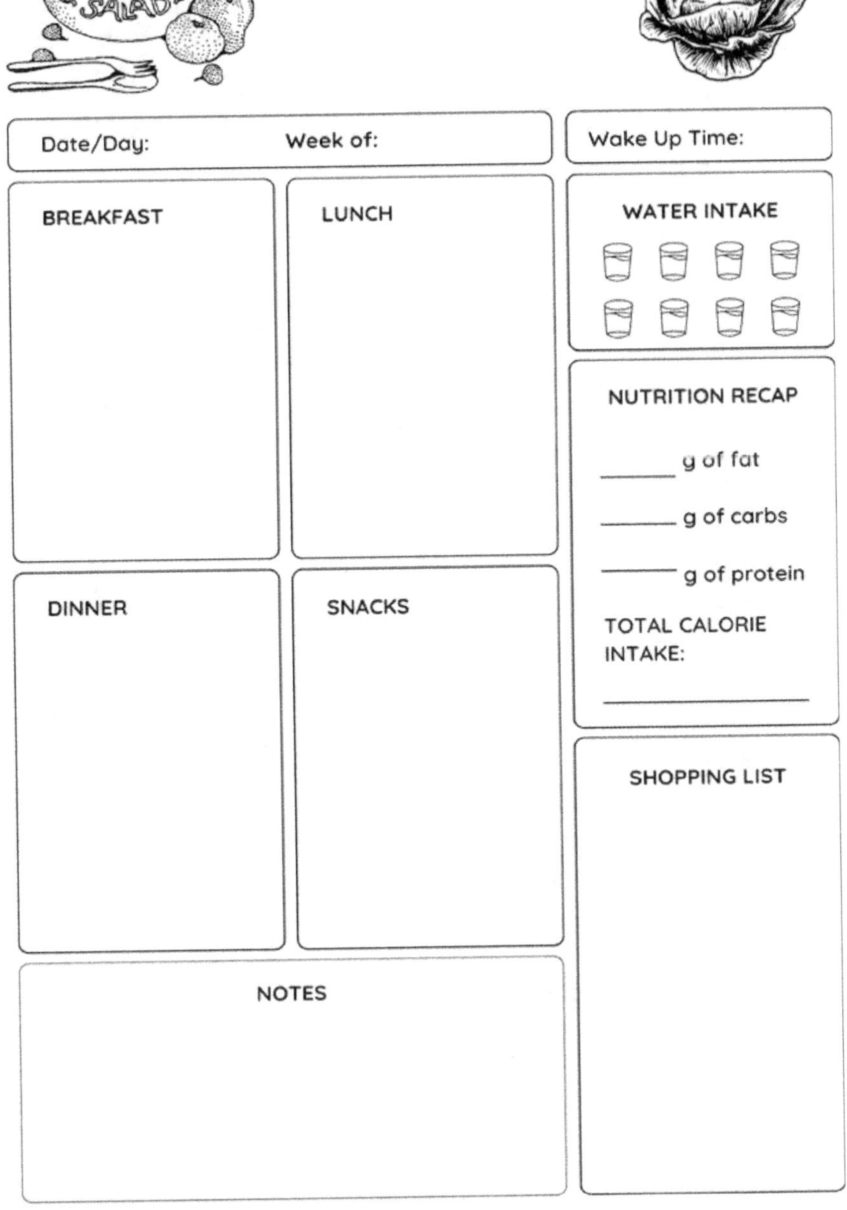

Date/Day:
Week of:
Wake Up Time:
BREAKFAST
LUNCH
WATER INTAKE
NUTRITION RECAP
_______ g of fat
_______ g of carbs
_______ g of protein
TOTAL CALORIE INTAKE:
DINNER
SNACKS
SHOPPING LIST
NOTES

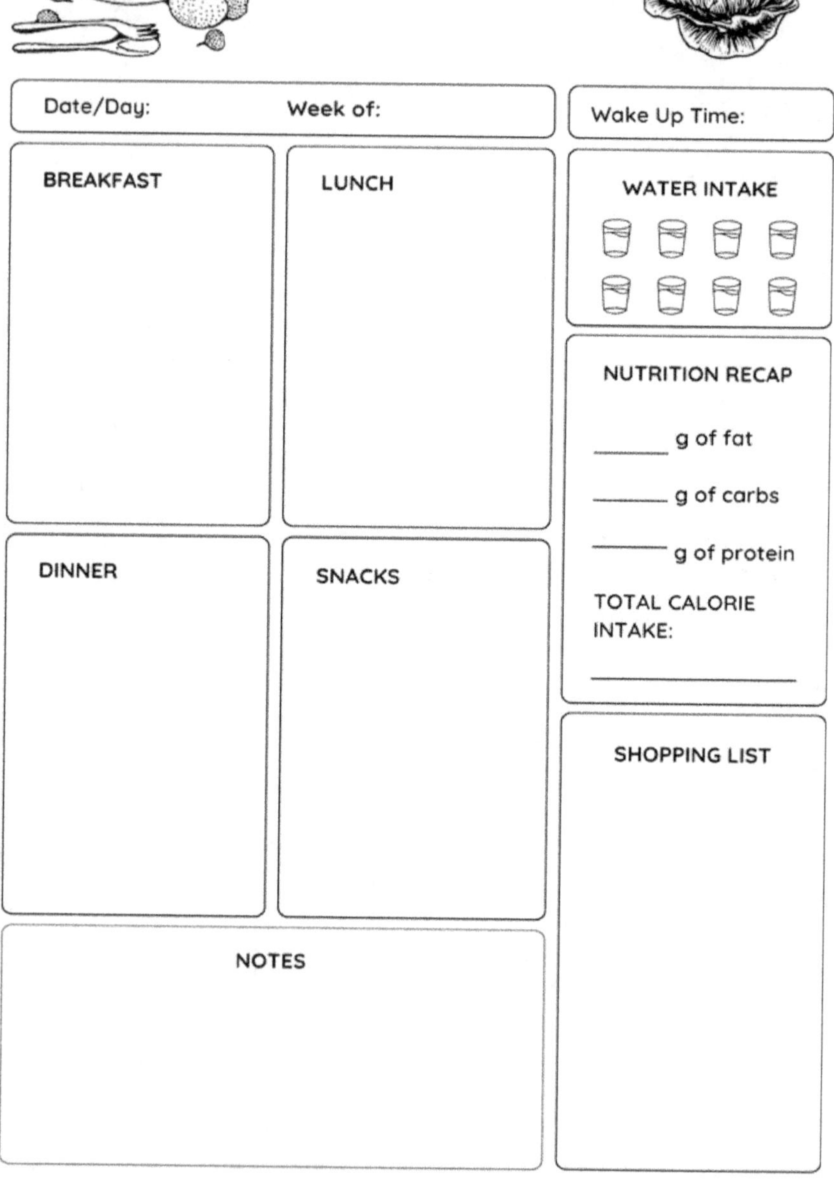

Date/Day: Week of:

Wake Up Time:

BREAKFAST

LUNCH

WATER INTAKE

NUTRITION RECAP

__________ g of fat

__________ g of carbs

__________ g of protein

TOTAL CALORIE INTAKE:

DINNER

SNACKS

SHOPPING LIST

NOTES

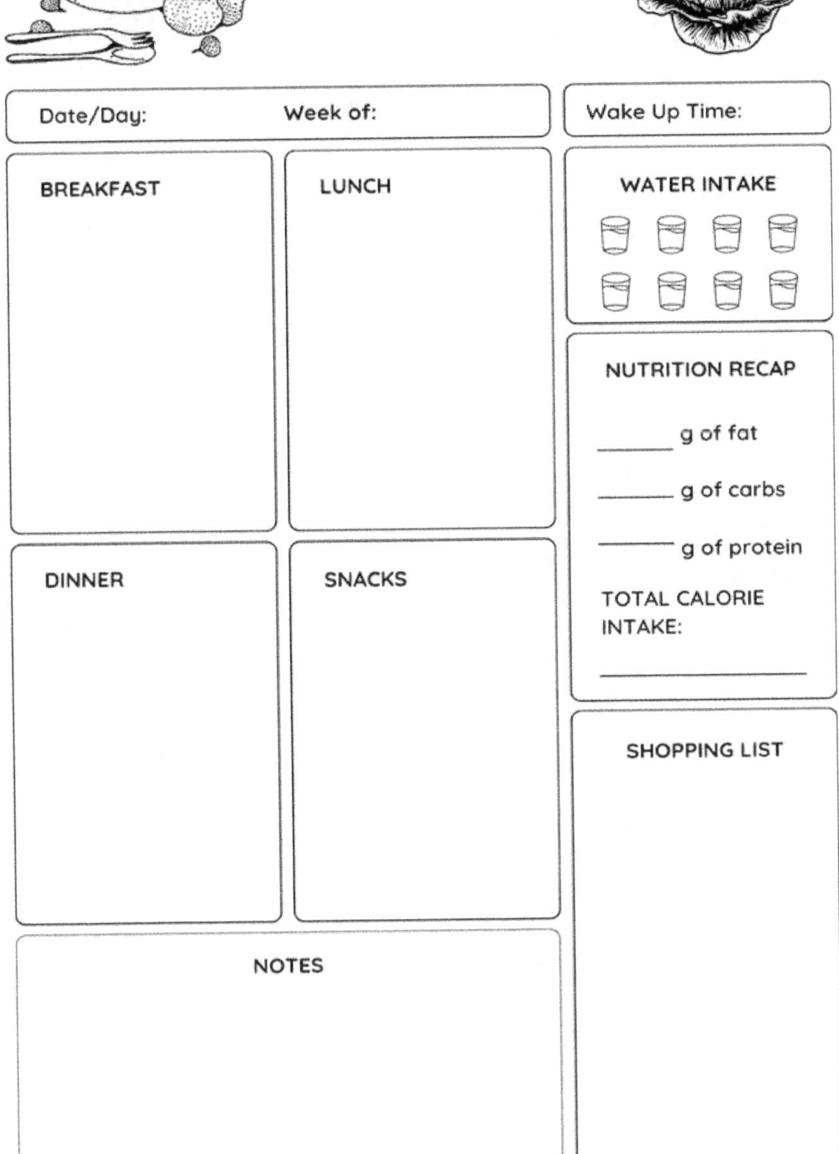

Date/Day:
Week of:
Wake Up Time:
BREAKFAST
LUNCH
WATER INTAKE
NUTRITION RECAP
_______ g of fat
_______ g of carbs
_______ g of protein
TOTAL CALORIE INTAKE:
DINNER
SNACKS
SHOPPING LIST
NOTES

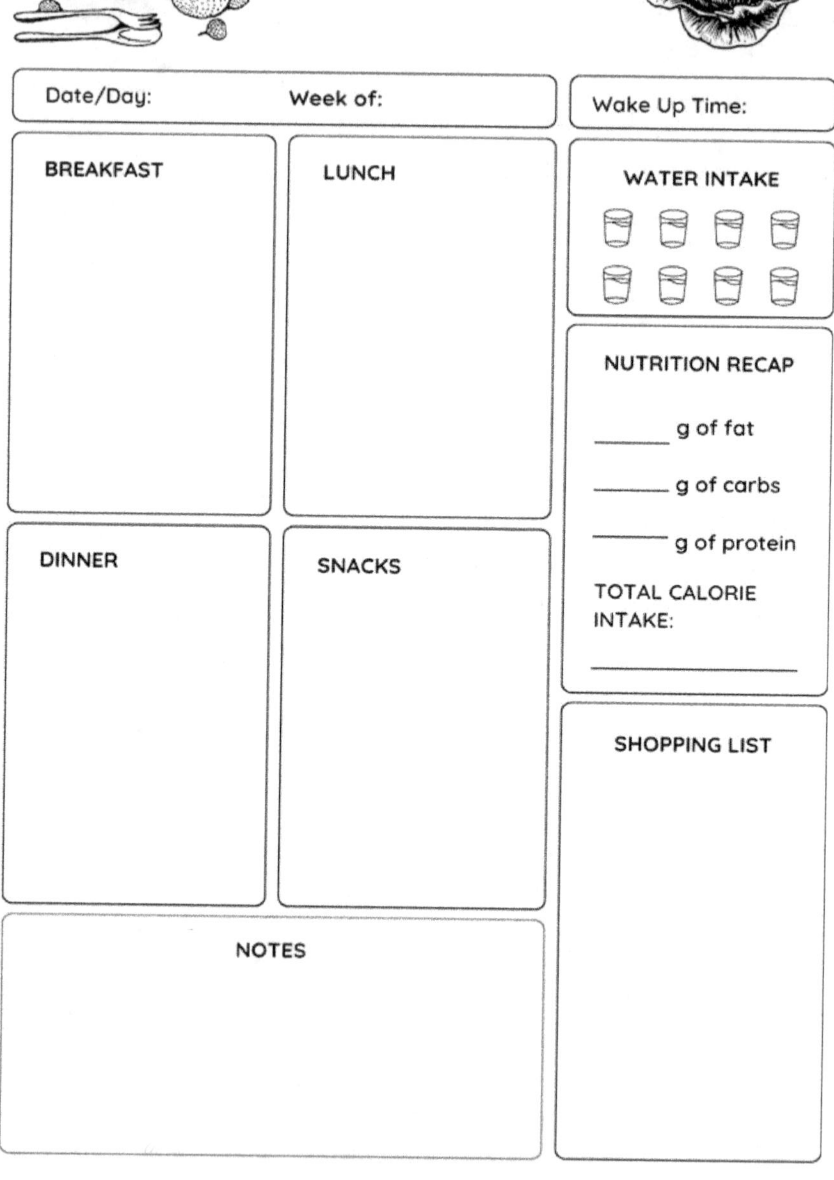

Date/Day:
Week of:
Wake Up Time:
BREAKFAST
LUNCH
WATER INTAKE
NUTRITION RECAP
_______ g of fat
_______ g of carbs
_______ g of protein
TOTAL CALORIE INTAKE:
DINNER
SNACKS
SHOPPING LIST
NOTES

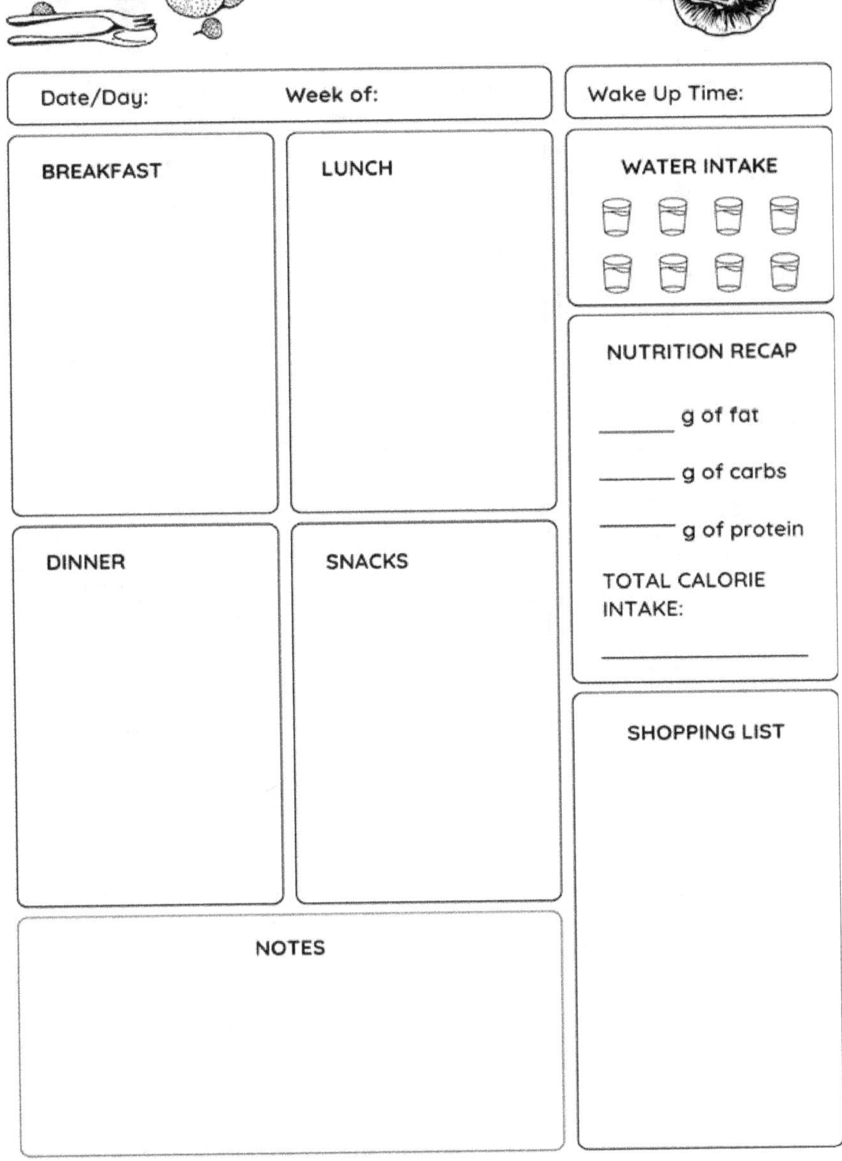

Date/Day:
Week of:
Wake Up Time:
BREAKFAST
LUNCH
WATER INTAKE
NUTRITION RECAP
_______ g of fat
_______ g of carbs
_______ g of protein
TOTAL CALORIE INTAKE:
DINNER
SNACKS
SHOPPING LIST
NOTES

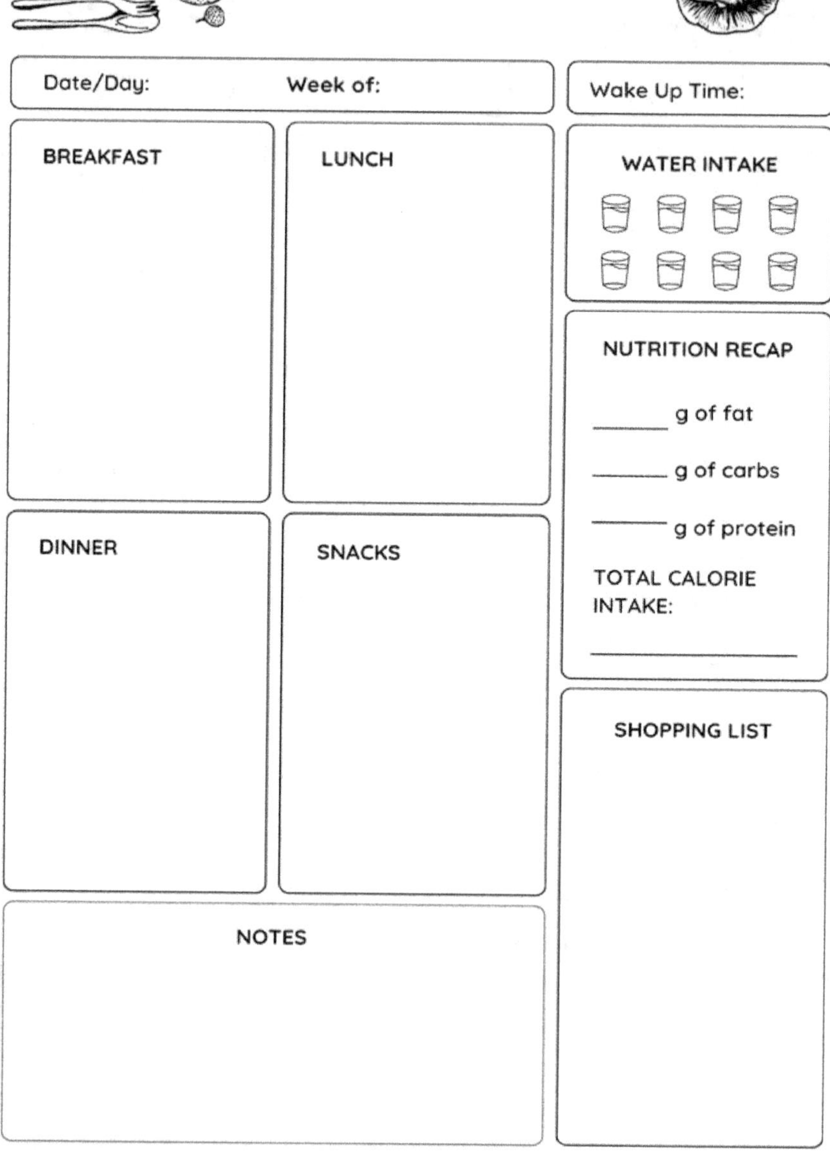

| Date/Day: | Week of: | Wake Up Time: |

BREAKFAST

LUNCH

WATER INTAKE

NUTRITION RECAP

_______ g of fat

_______ g of carbs

_______ g of protein

TOTAL CALORIE INTAKE:

DINNER

SNACKS

SHOPPING LIST

NOTES

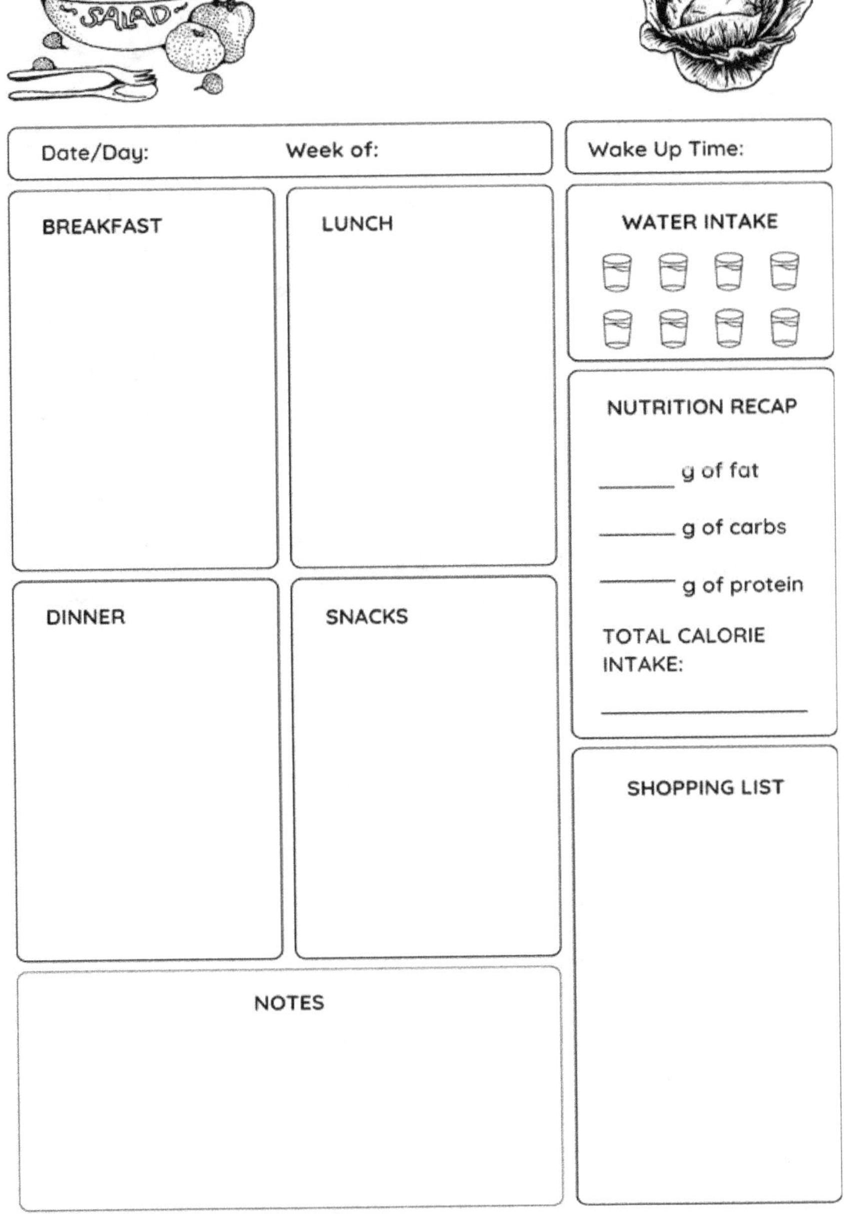

Date/Day: Week of:

Wake Up Time:

BREAKFAST

LUNCH

WATER INTAKE

NUTRITION RECAP

_______ g of fat

_______ g of carbs

_______ g of protein

TOTAL CALORIE
INTAKE:

____

DINNER

SNACKS

SHOPPING LIST

NOTES

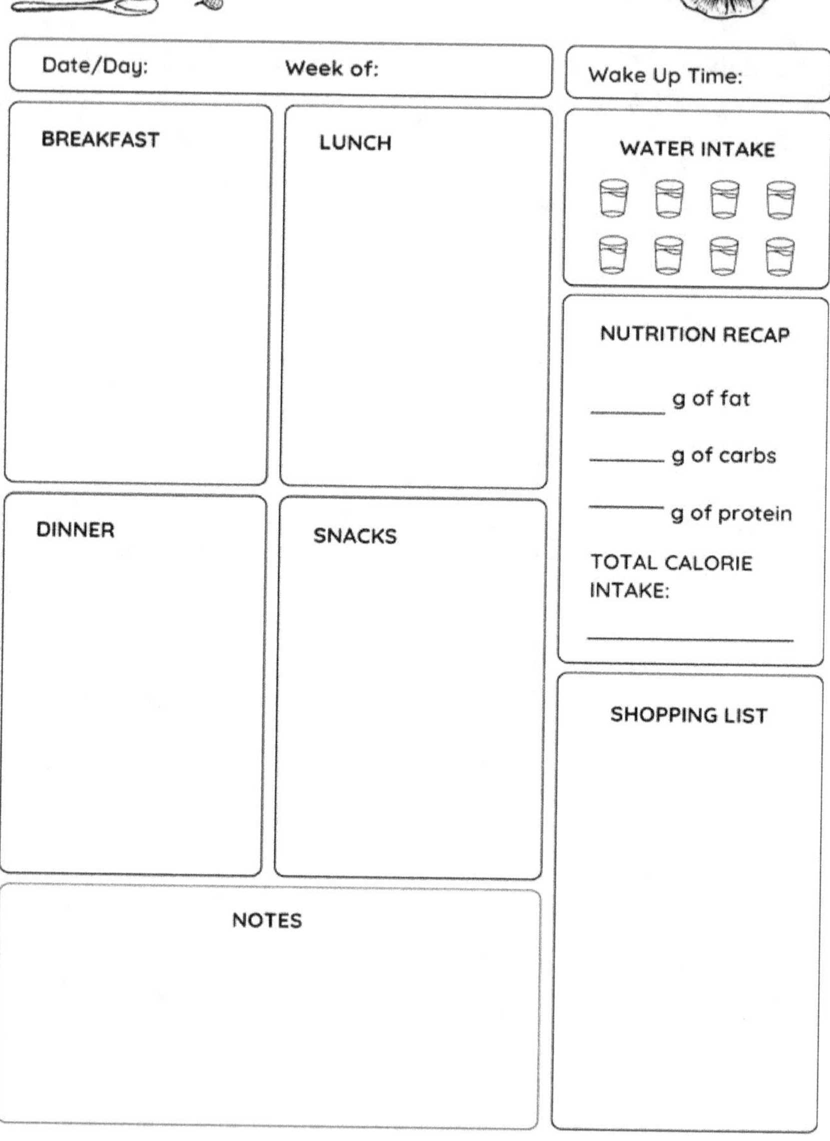

Date/Day: Week of:

Wake Up Time:

BREAKFAST

LUNCH

WATER INTAKE

NUTRITION RECAP

_______ g of fat

_______ g of carbs

_______ g of protein

TOTAL CALORIE INTAKE:

____

DINNER

SNACKS

SHOPPING LIST

NOTES

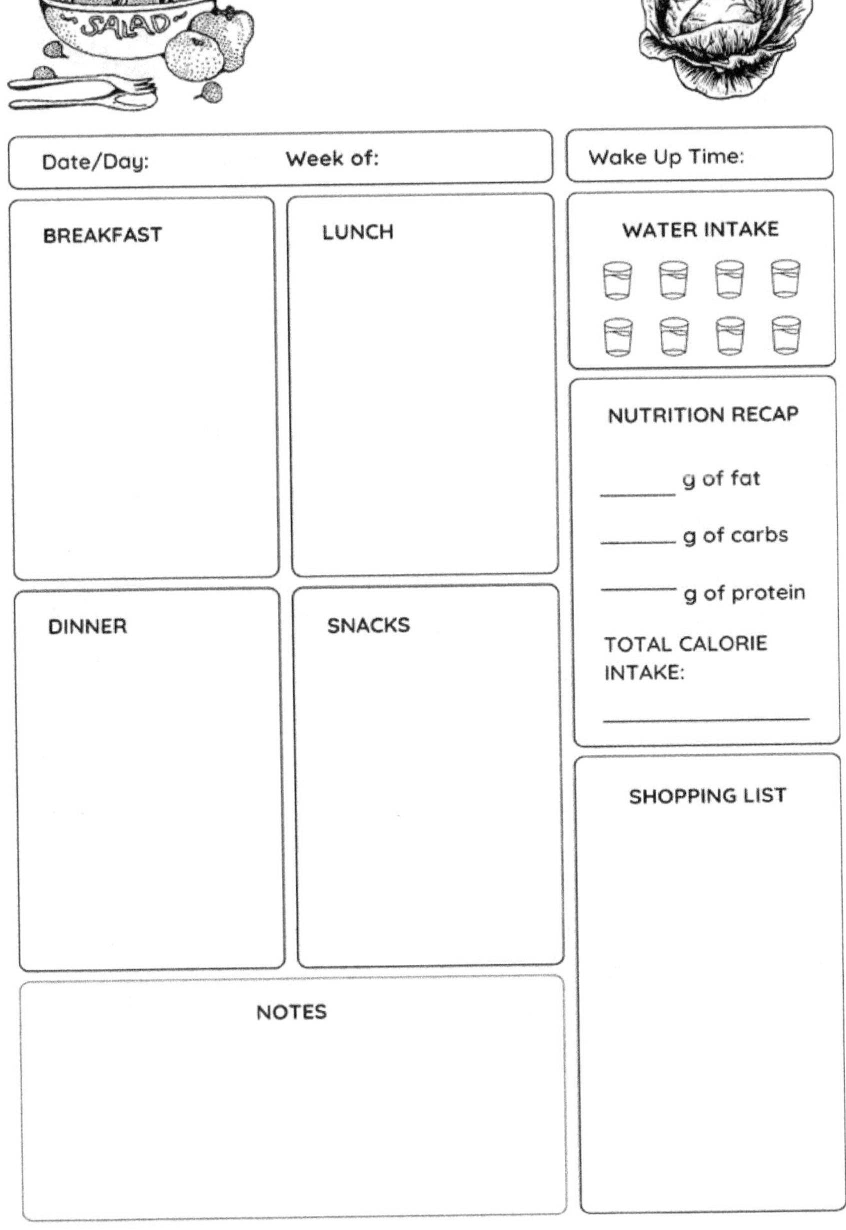

Date/Day: | Week of:

Wake Up Time:

BREAKFAST

LUNCH

WATER INTAKE

NUTRITION RECAP

_______ g of fat

_______ g of carbs

_______ g of protein

TOTAL CALORIE INTAKE:

____

DINNER

SNACKS

SHOPPING LIST

NOTES

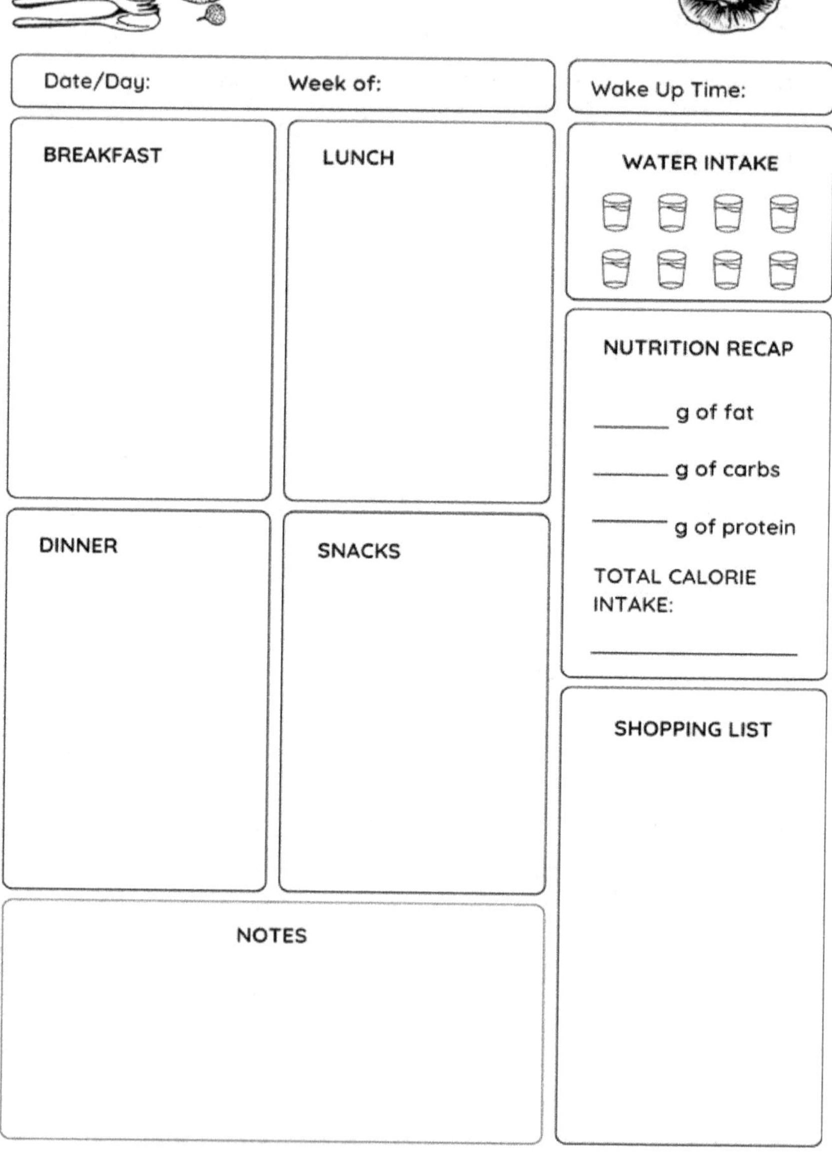

Date/Day: Week of:

Wake Up Time:

BREAKFAST

LUNCH

WATER INTAKE

NUTRITION RECAP

_______ g of fat

_______ g of carbs

_______ g of protein

TOTAL CALORIE INTAKE:

____

DINNER

SNACKS

SHOPPING LIST

NOTES

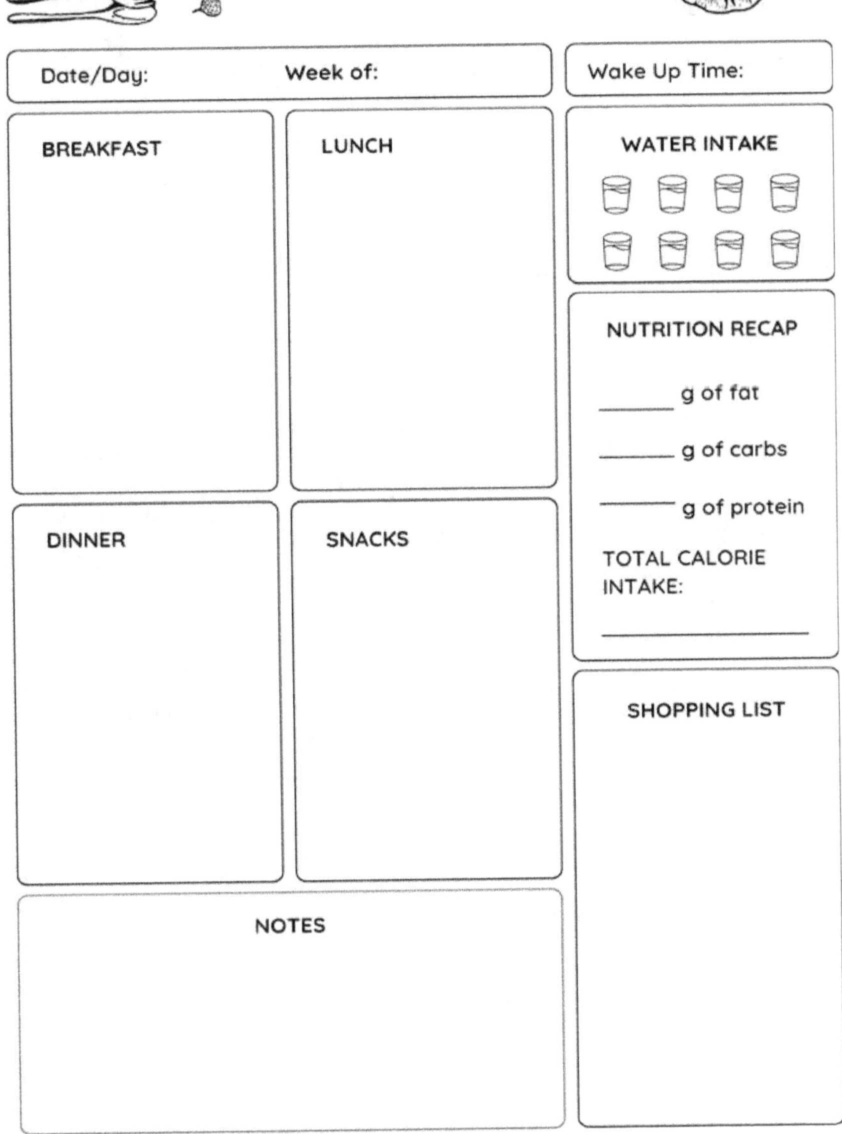

Date/Day:
Week of:
Wake Up Time:
BREAKFAST
LUNCH
WATER INTAKE
NUTRITION RECAP
_______ g of fat
_______ g of carbs
_______ g of protein
TOTAL CALORIE INTAKE:
DINNER
SNACKS
SHOPPING LIST
NOTES

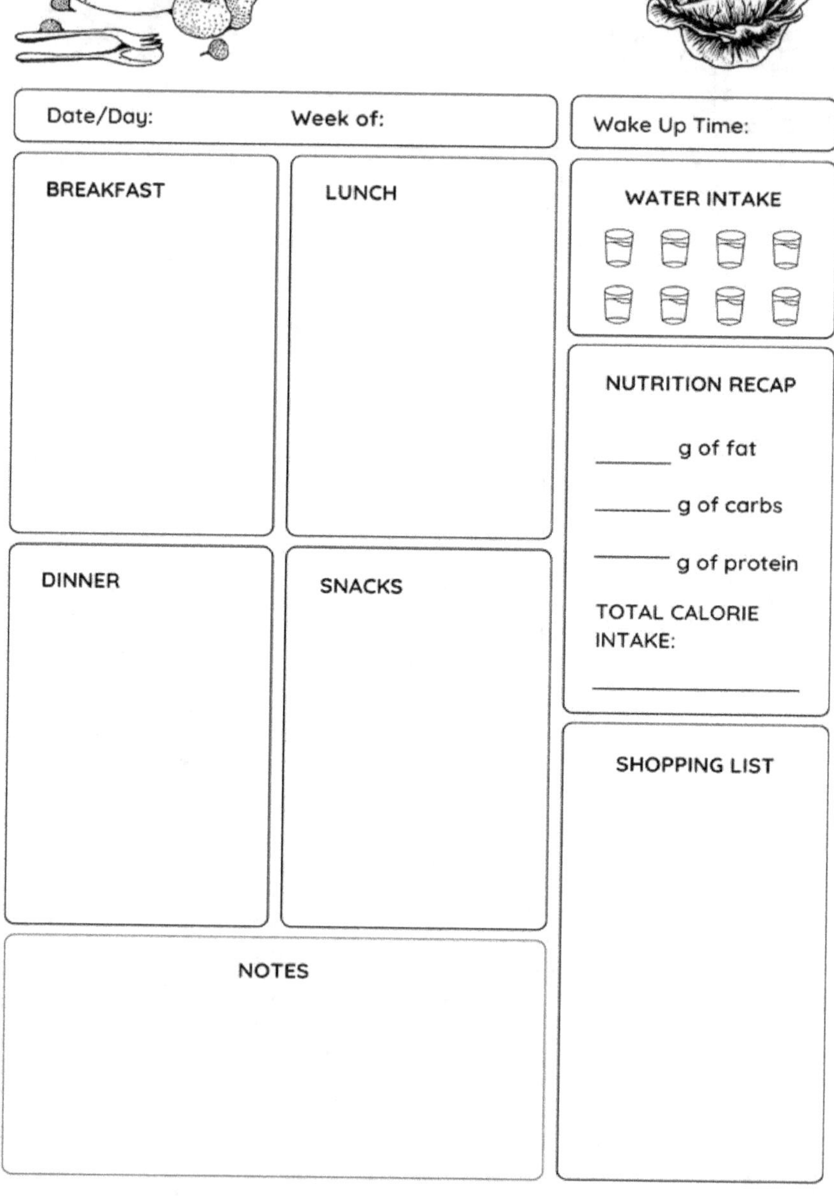

Date/Day:
Week of:
Wake Up Time:
BREAKFAST
LUNCH
WATER INTAKE
NUTRITION RECAP
_______ g of fat
_______ g of carbs
_______ g of protein
TOTAL CALORIE INTAKE:
DINNER
SNACKS
SHOPPING LIST
NOTES

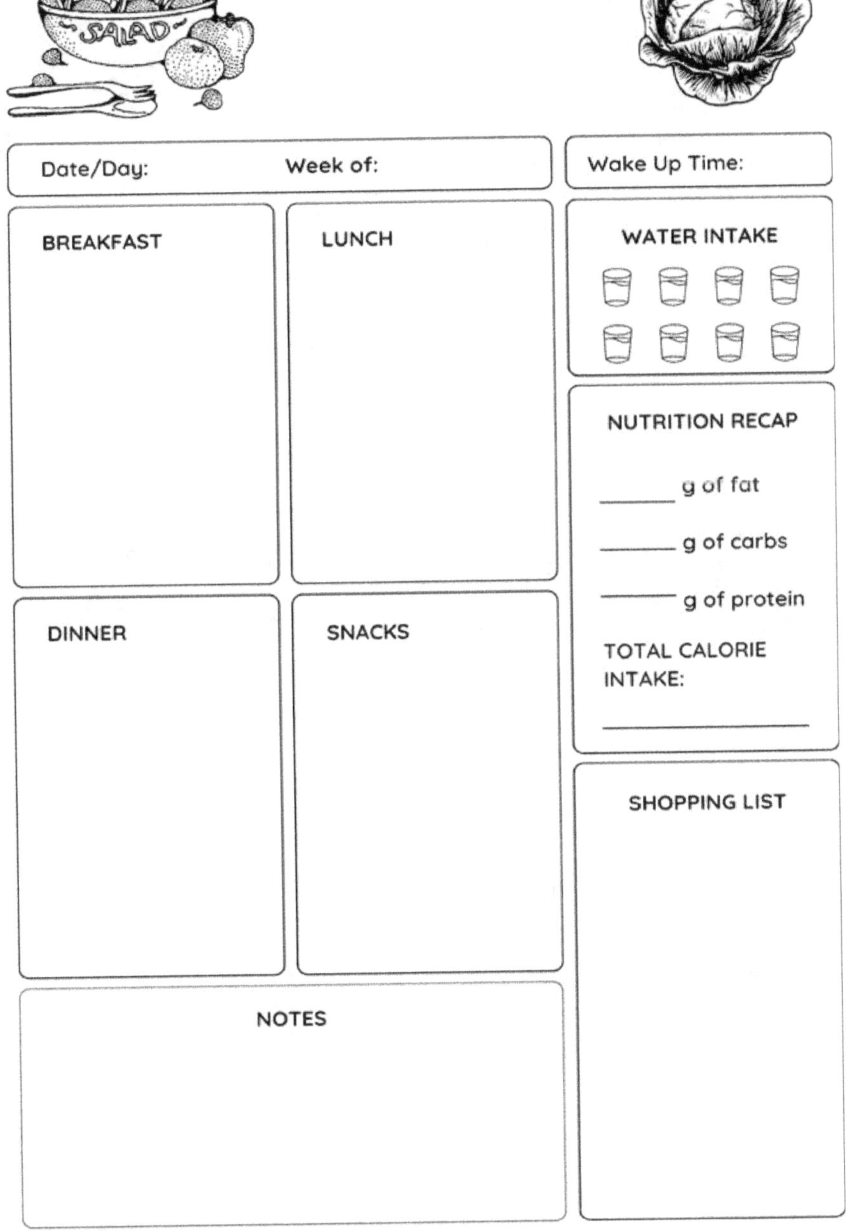

| Date/Day: | Week of: | Wake Up Time: |

BREAKFAST

LUNCH

WATER INTAKE

NUTRITION RECAP

__________ g of fat

__________ g of carbs

__________ g of protein

TOTAL CALORIE INTAKE:

DINNER

SNACKS

SHOPPING LIST

NOTES

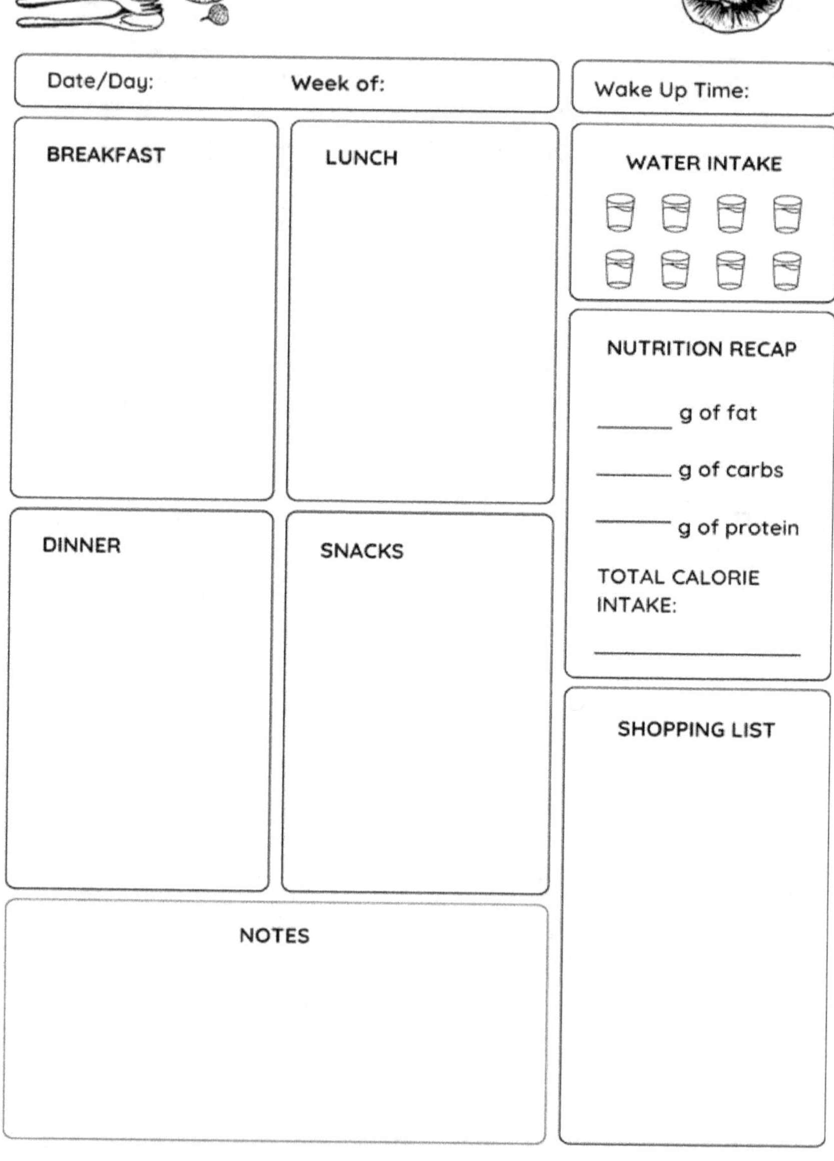

| Date/Day: | Week of: | Wake Up Time: |

BREAKFAST

LUNCH

WATER INTAKE

NUTRITION RECAP

_______ g of fat

_______ g of carbs

_______ g of protein

TOTAL CALORIE INTAKE:

____

DINNER

SNACKS

SHOPPING LIST

NOTES

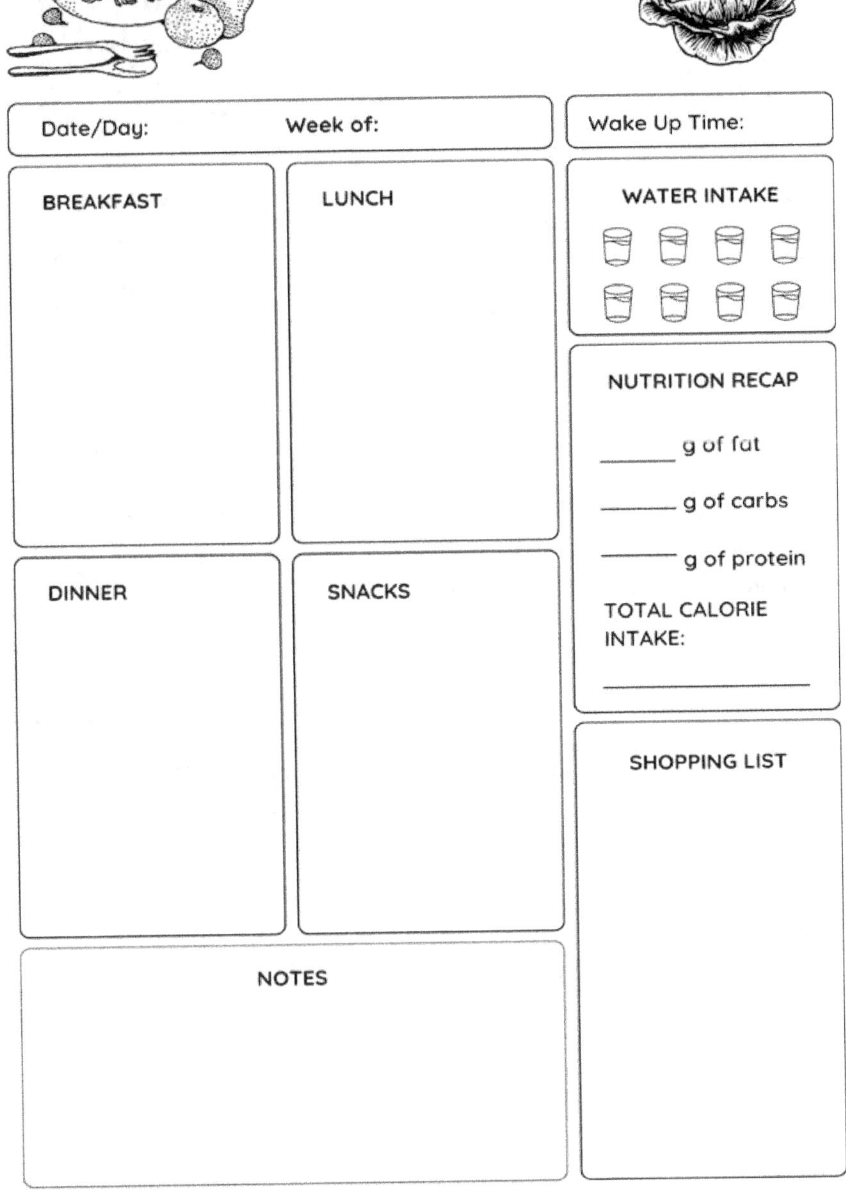

Date/Day: Week of:

Wake Up Time:

BREAKFAST

LUNCH

WATER INTAKE

NUTRITION RECAP

_______ g of fat

_______ g of carbs

_______ g of protein

TOTAL CALORIE INTAKE:

____

DINNER

SNACKS

SHOPPING LIST

NOTES

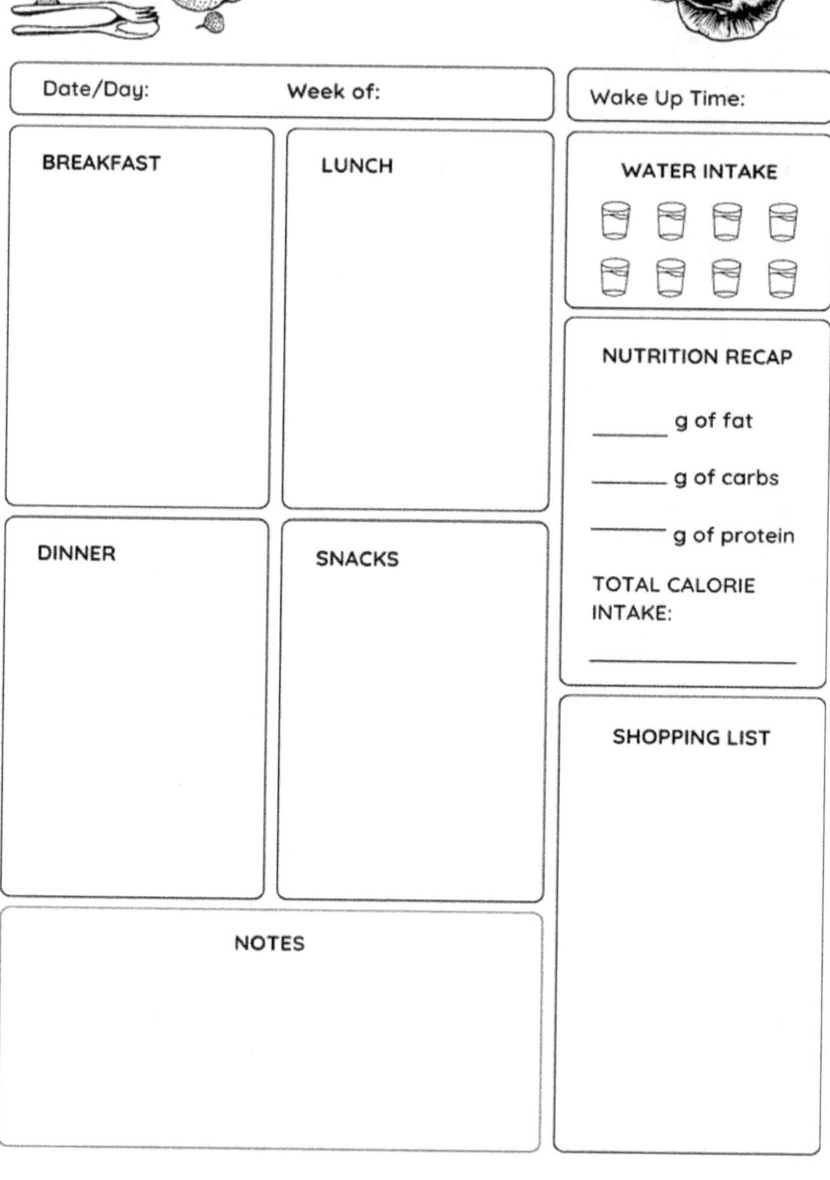

Date/Day:
Week of:
Wake Up Time:
BREAKFAST
LUNCH
WATER INTAKE
NUTRITION RECAP
_______ g of fat
_______ g of carbs
_______ g of protein
TOTAL CALORIE INTAKE:
DINNER
SNACKS
SHOPPING LIST
NOTES

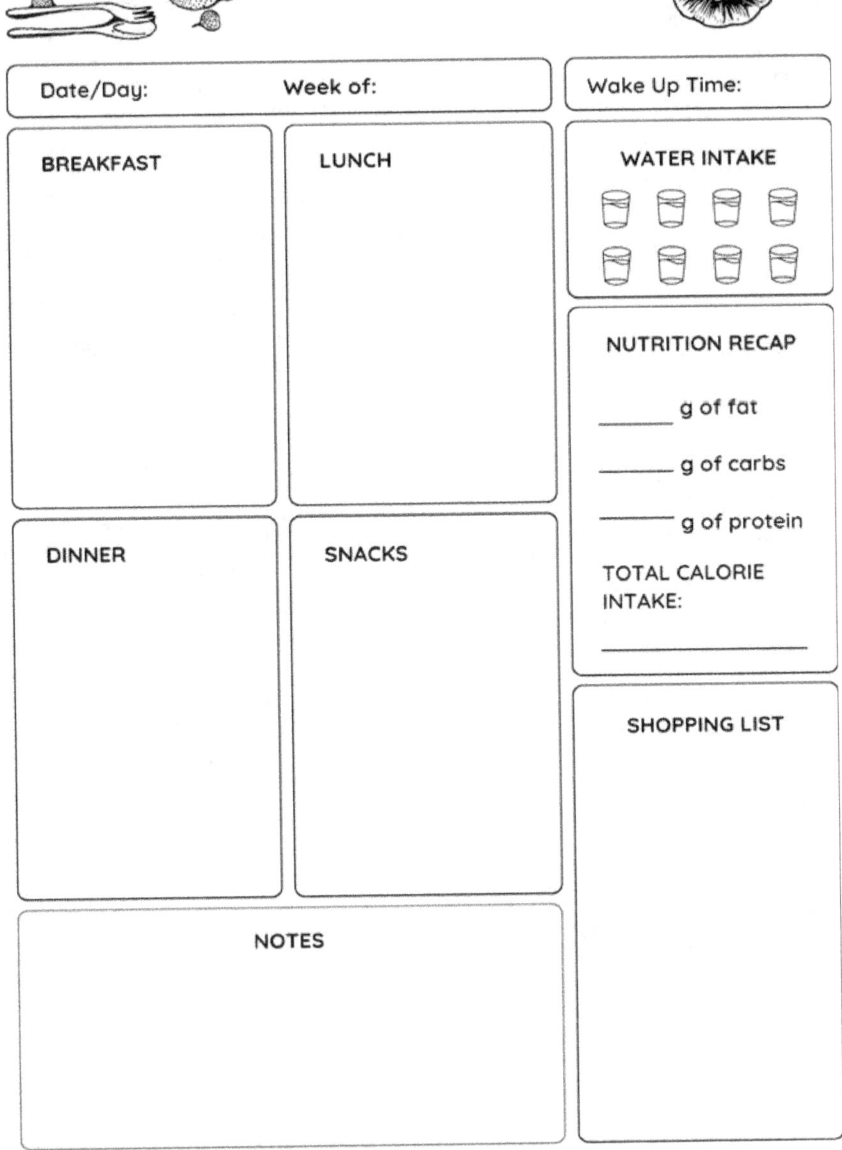

Date/Day: Week of:

Wake Up Time:

BREAKFAST

LUNCH

WATER INTAKE

NUTRITION RECAP

_______ g of fat

_______ g of carbs

_______ g of protein

TOTAL CALORIE INTAKE:

____

DINNER

SNACKS

SHOPPING LIST

NOTES

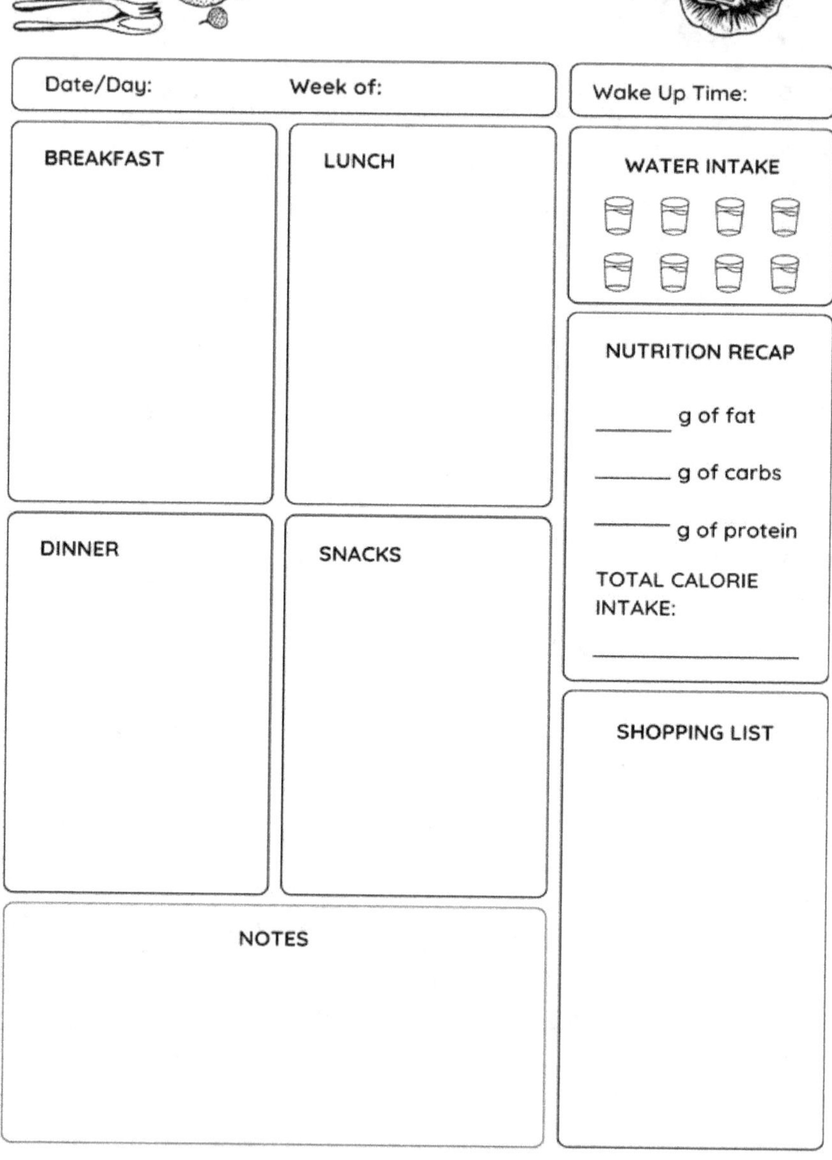

Date/Day: Week of:
Wake Up Time:

BREAKFAST

LUNCH

WATER INTAKE

NUTRITION RECAP

_______ g of fat

_______ g of carbs

_______ g of protein

TOTAL CALORIE INTAKE:

DINNER

SNACKS

SHOPPING LIST

NOTES

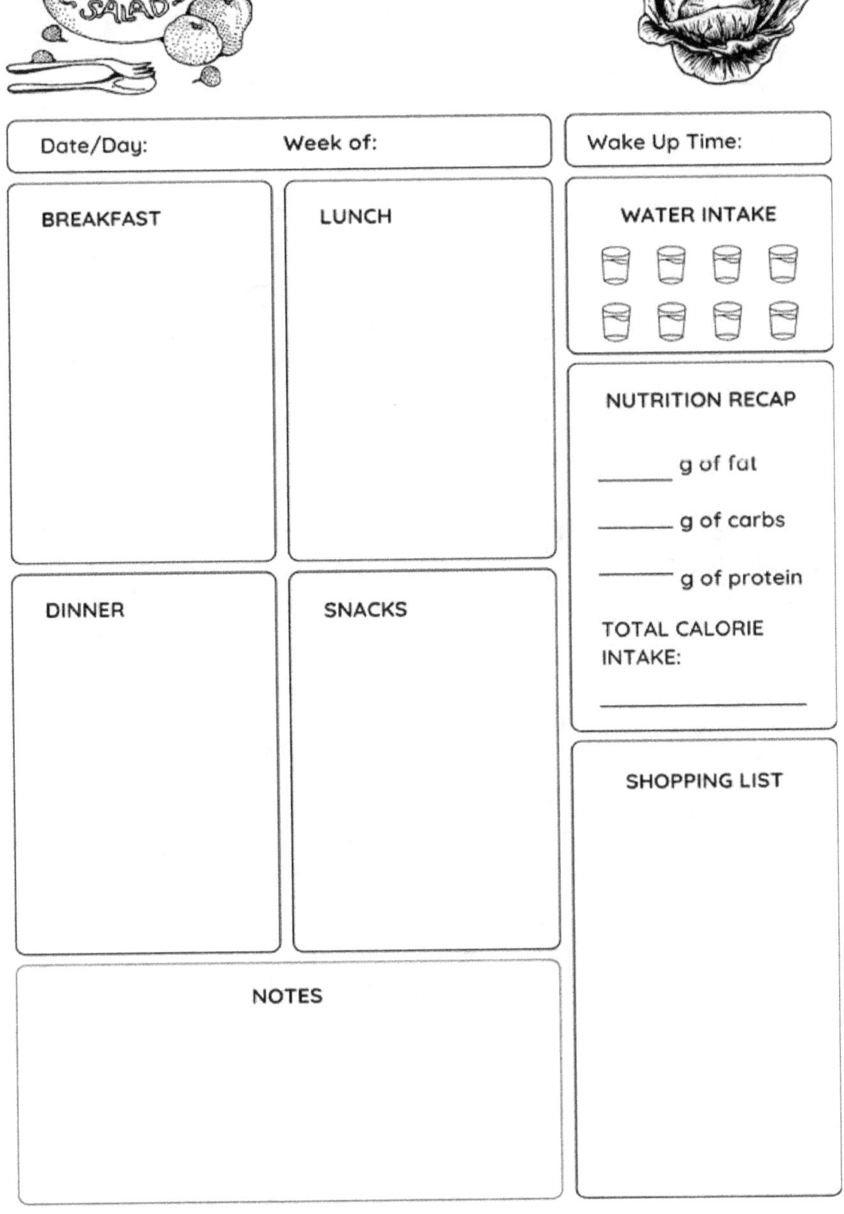

Date/Day: Week of:

Wake Up Time:

BREAKFAST

LUNCH

WATER INTAKE

NUTRITION RECAP

_______ g of fat

_______ g of carbs

_______ g of protein

TOTAL CALORIE INTAKE:

____

DINNER

SNACKS

SHOPPING LIST

NOTES

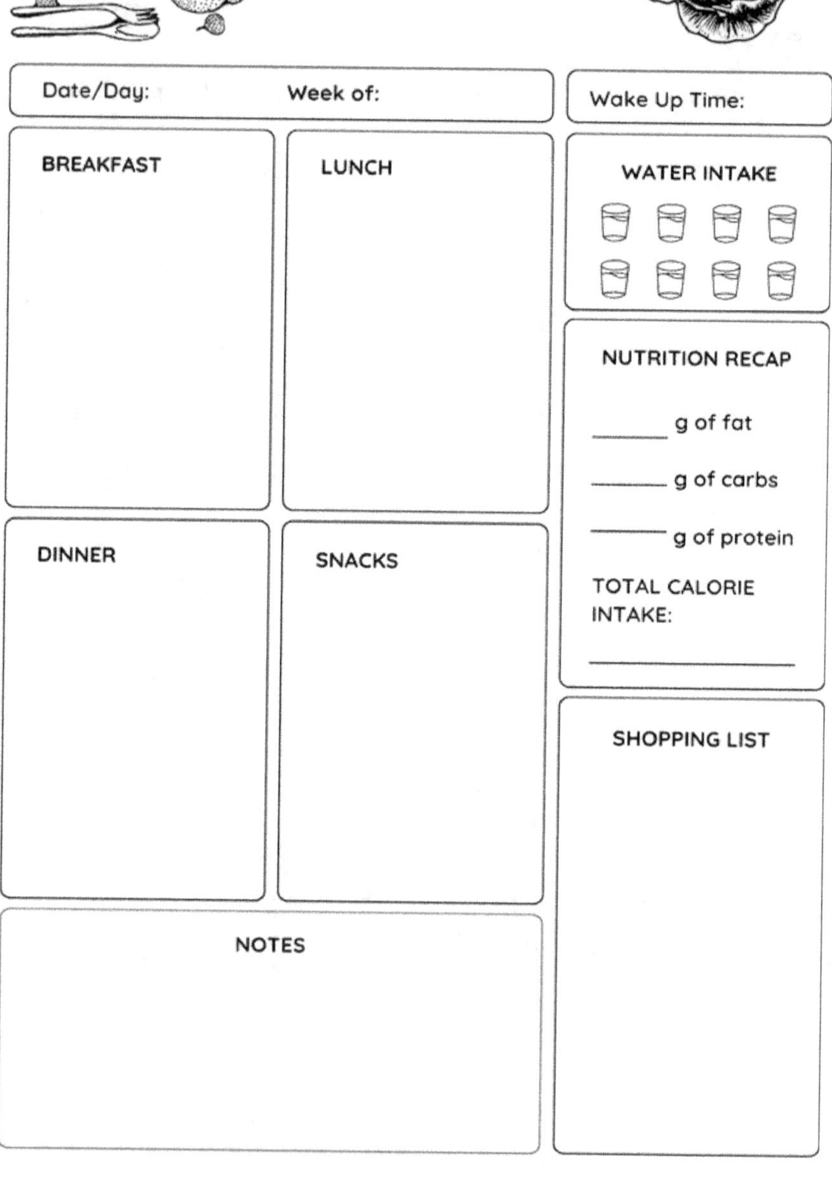

Date/Day: Week of:

Wake Up Time:

BREAKFAST

LUNCH

WATER INTAKE

NUTRITION RECAP

________ g of fat

________ g of carbs

________ g of protein

TOTAL CALORIE INTAKE:

____

DINNER

SNACKS

SHOPPING LIST

NOTES

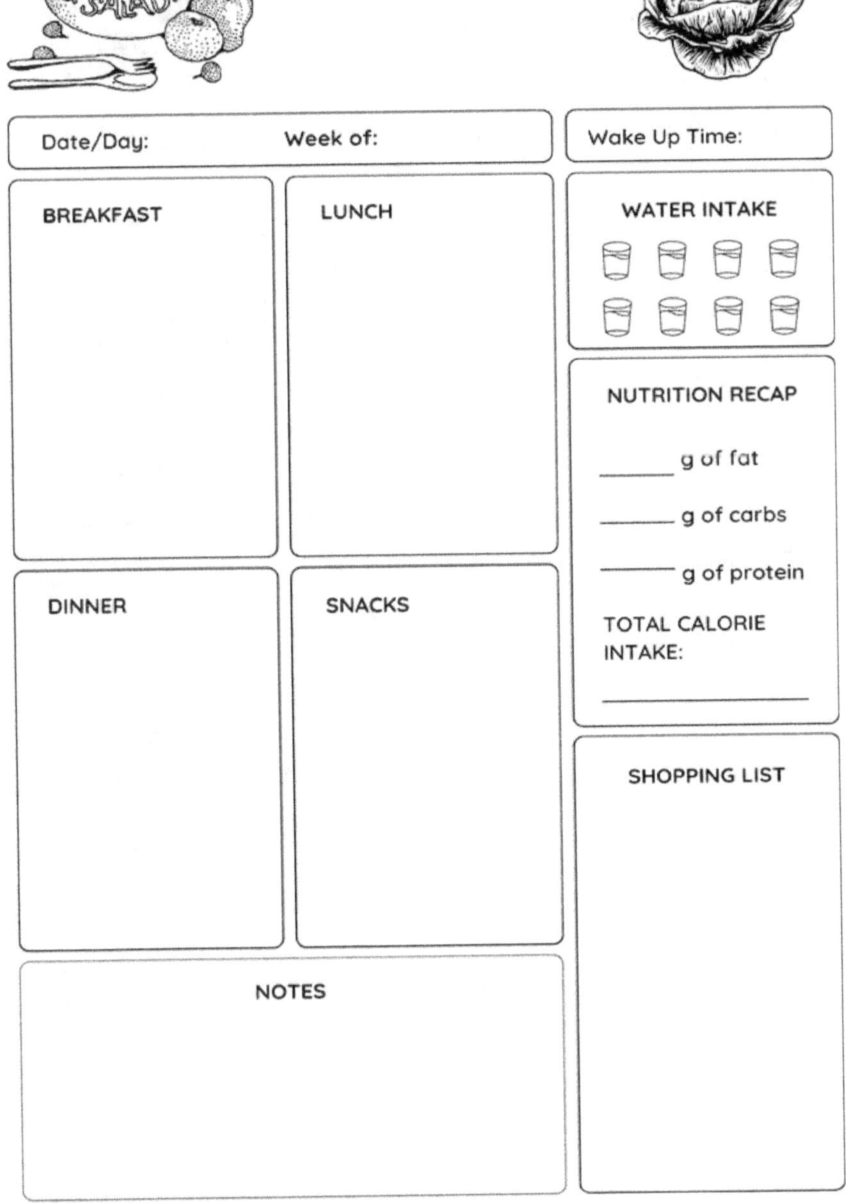

Date/Day: Week of:

Wake Up Time:

BREAKFAST

LUNCH

WATER INTAKE

NUTRITION RECAP

______ g of fat

______ g of carbs

______ g of protein

TOTAL CALORIE INTAKE:

DINNER

SNACKS

SHOPPING LIST

NOTES

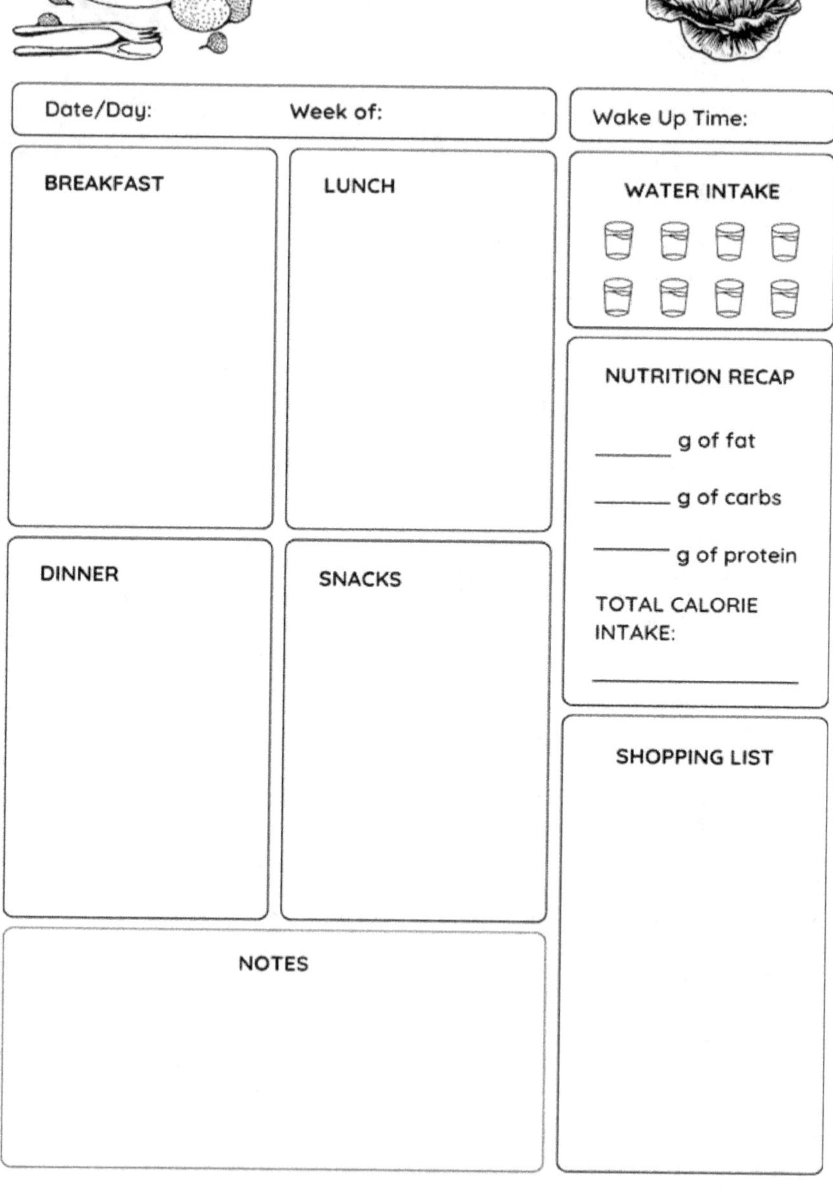

Date/Day:
Week of:
Wake Up Time:
BREAKFAST
LUNCH
WATER INTAKE
NUTRITION RECAP
_______ g of fat
_______ g of carbs
_______ g of protein
TOTAL CALORIE INTAKE:
DINNER
SNACKS
SHOPPING LIST
NOTES

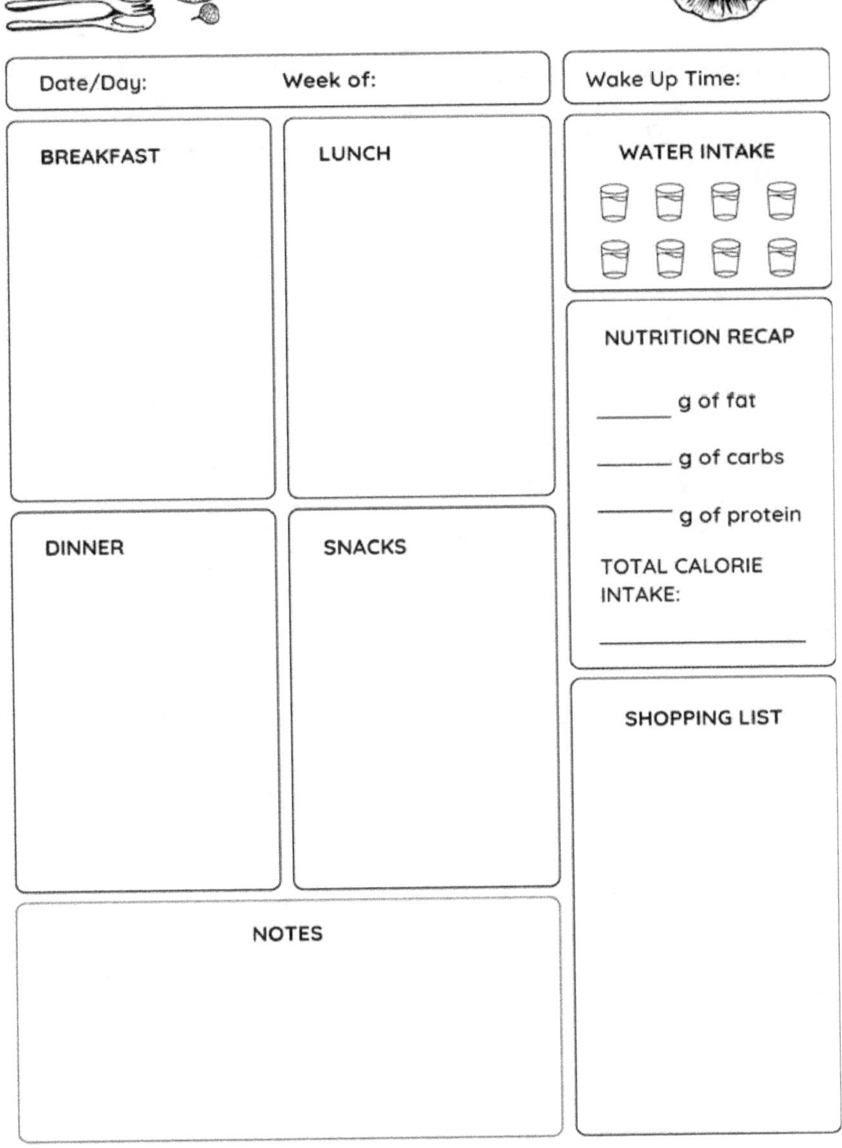

Date/Day: Week of:

Wake Up Time:

BREAKFAST

LUNCH

WATER INTAKE

NUTRITION RECAP

_______ g of fat

_______ g of carbs

_______ g of protein

TOTAL CALORIE INTAKE:

DINNER

SNACKS

SHOPPING LIST

NOTES

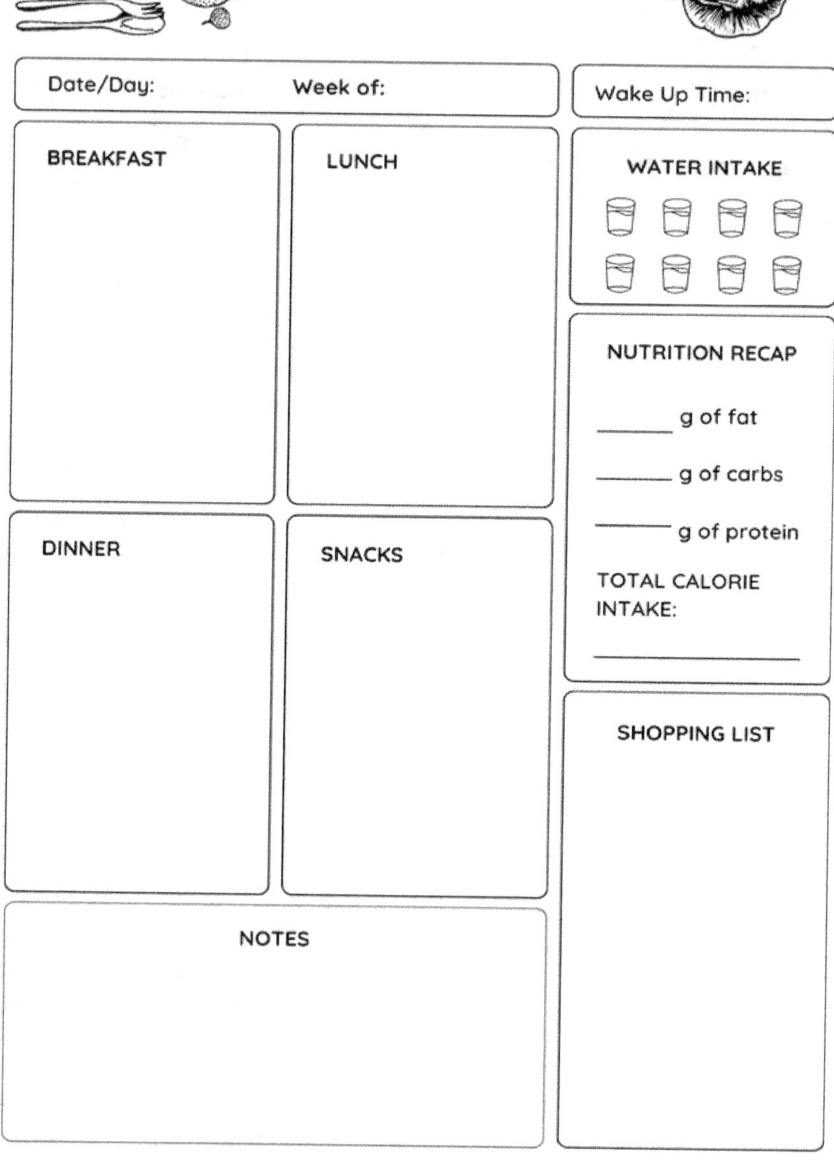

| Date/Day: | Week of: | | Wake Up Time: |

BREAKFAST

LUNCH

WATER INTAKE

NUTRITION RECAP

______ g of fat

______ g of carbs

______ g of protein

TOTAL CALORIE INTAKE:

DINNER

SNACKS

SHOPPING LIST

NOTES

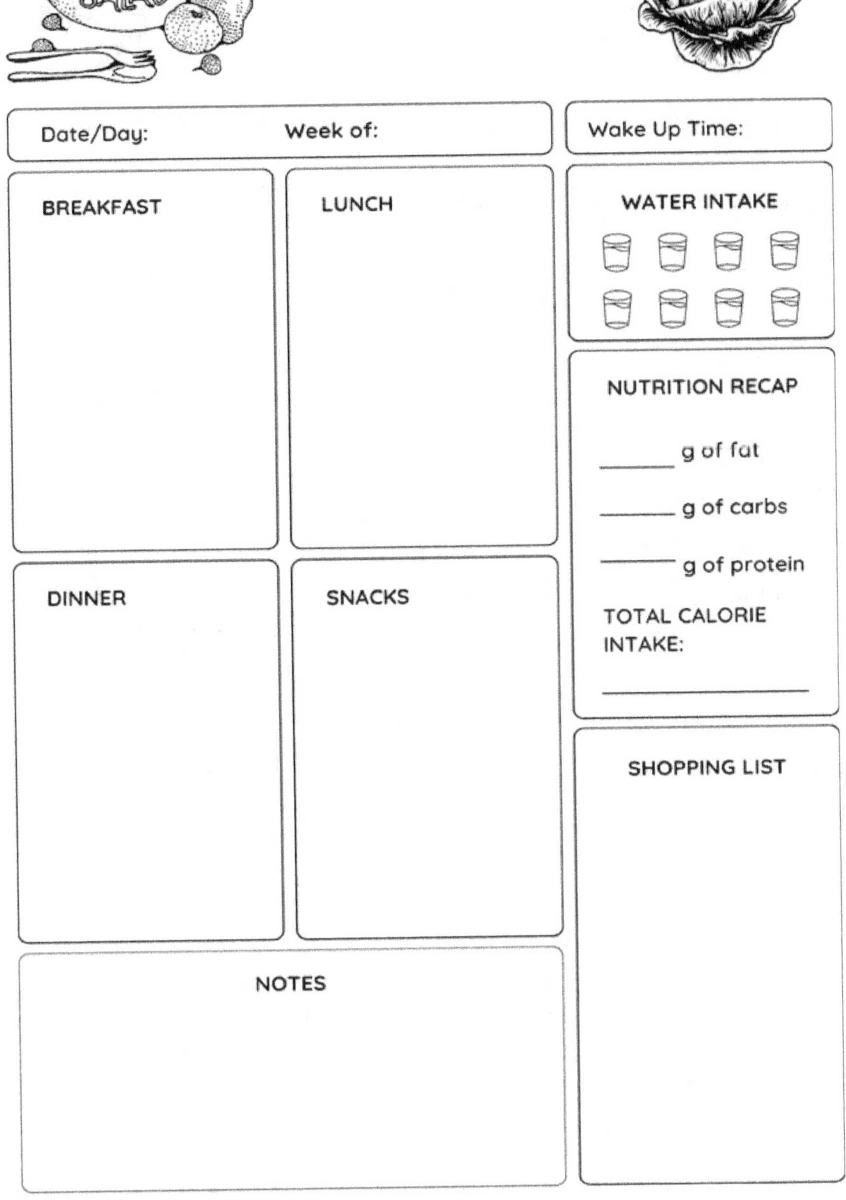

Date/Day: Week of:

Wake Up Time:

BREAKFAST

LUNCH

WATER INTAKE

NUTRITION RECAP

_______ g of fat

_______ g of carbs

_______ g of protein

TOTAL CALORIE INTAKE:

____

DINNER

SNACKS

SHOPPING LIST

NOTES

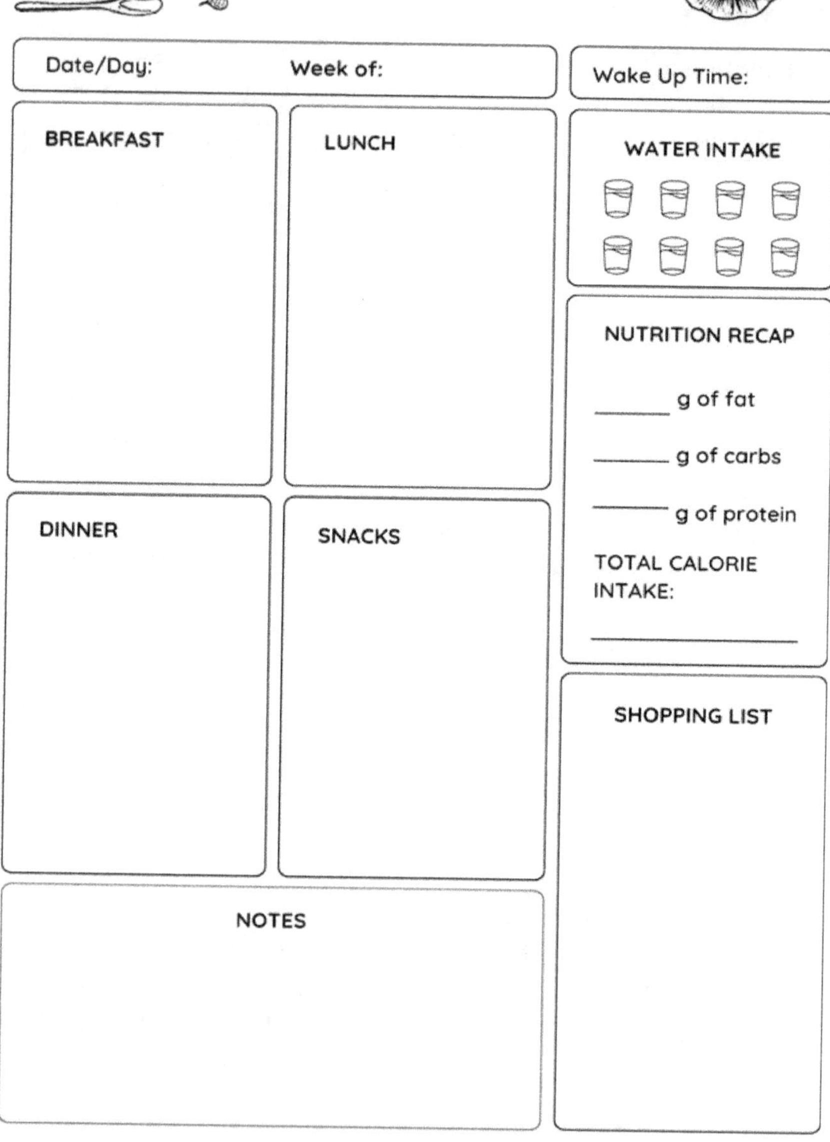

Date/Day: Week of:

Wake Up Time:

BREAKFAST

LUNCH

WATER INTAKE

NUTRITION RECAP

__________ g of fat

__________ g of carbs

__________ g of protein

TOTAL CALORIE INTAKE:

____

DINNER

SNACKS

SHOPPING LIST

NOTES

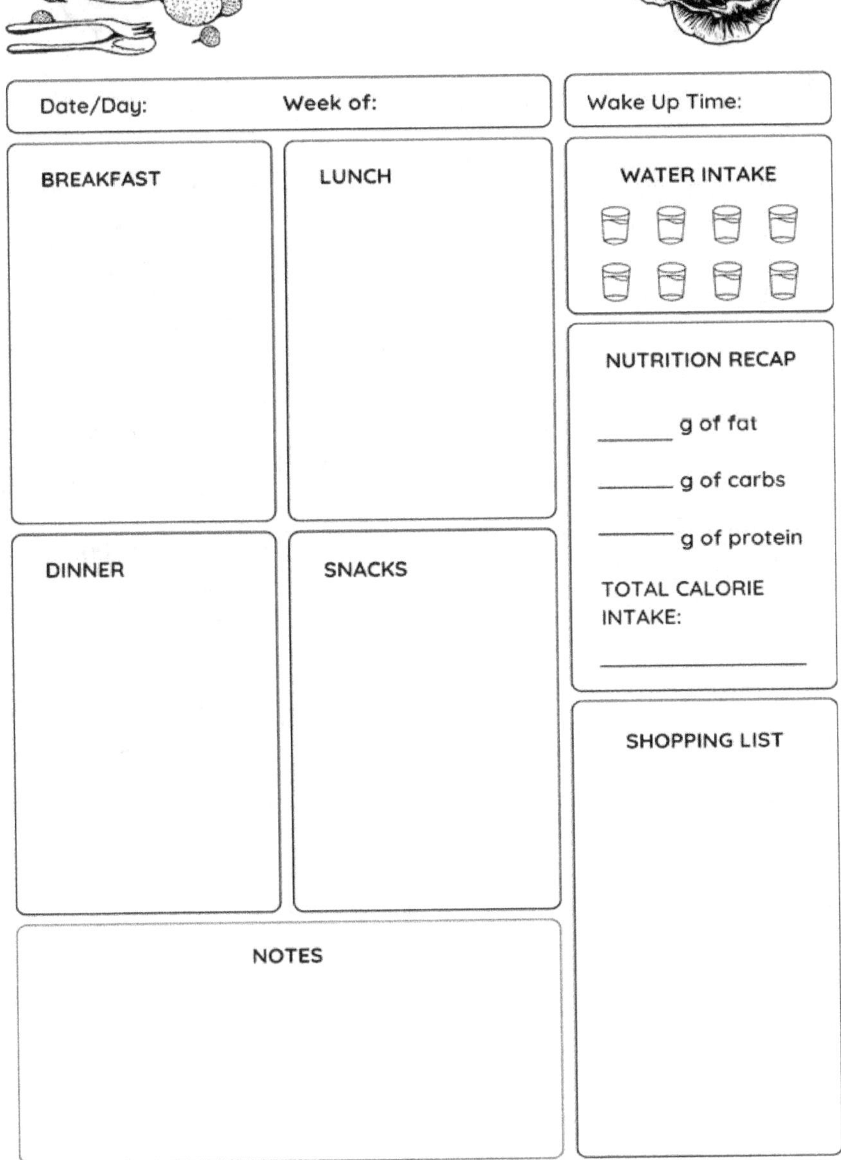

| Date/Day: | Week of: | Wake Up Time: |

BREAKFAST

LUNCH

WATER INTAKE

NUTRITION RECAP

_______ g of fat

_______ g of carbs

_______ g of protein

TOTAL CALORIE INTAKE:

____

DINNER

SNACKS

SHOPPING LIST

NOTES

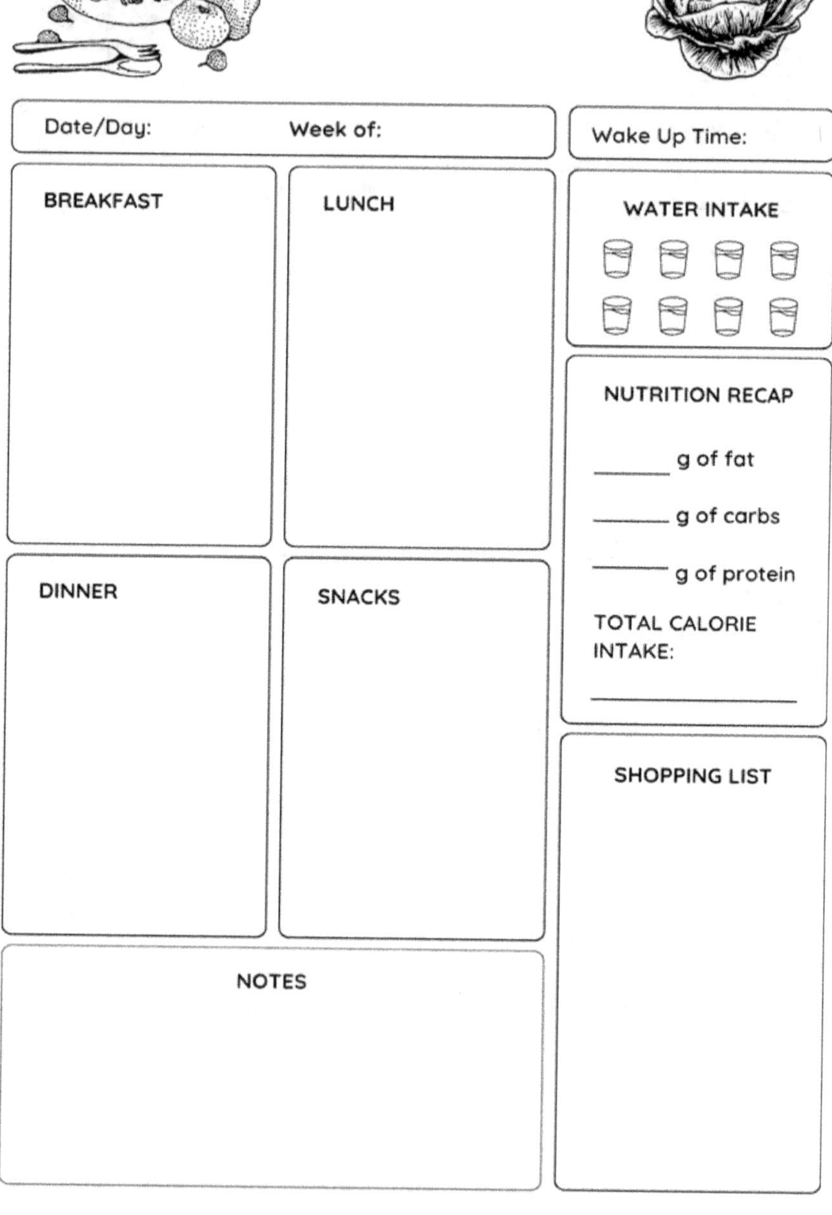

Date/Day: Week of:

Wake Up Time:

BREAKFAST

LUNCH

WATER INTAKE

NUTRITION RECAP

__________ g of fat

__________ g of carbs

__________ g of protein

TOTAL CALORIE INTAKE:

____

DINNER

SNACKS

SHOPPING LIST

NOTES

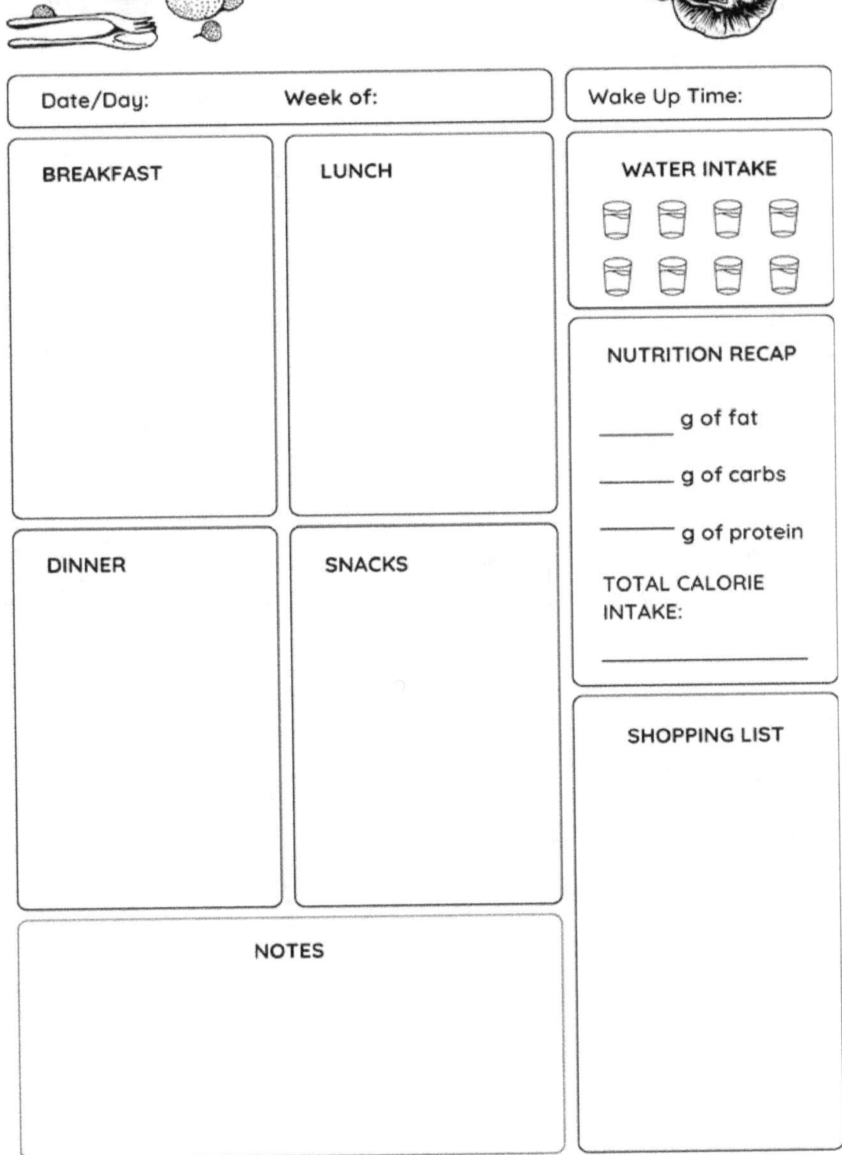

<table>
<tr><td colspan="2">Date/Day: Week of:</td><td>Wake Up Time:</td></tr>
<tr><td>BREAKFAST</td><td>LUNCH</td><td>WATER INTAKE</td></tr>
<tr><td>DINNER</td><td>SNACKS</td><td>NUTRITION RECAP

_______ g of fat

_______ g of carbs

_______ g of protein

TOTAL CALORIE INTAKE:

_______________</td></tr>
<tr><td colspan="2">NOTES</td><td>SHOPPING LIST</td></tr>
</table>

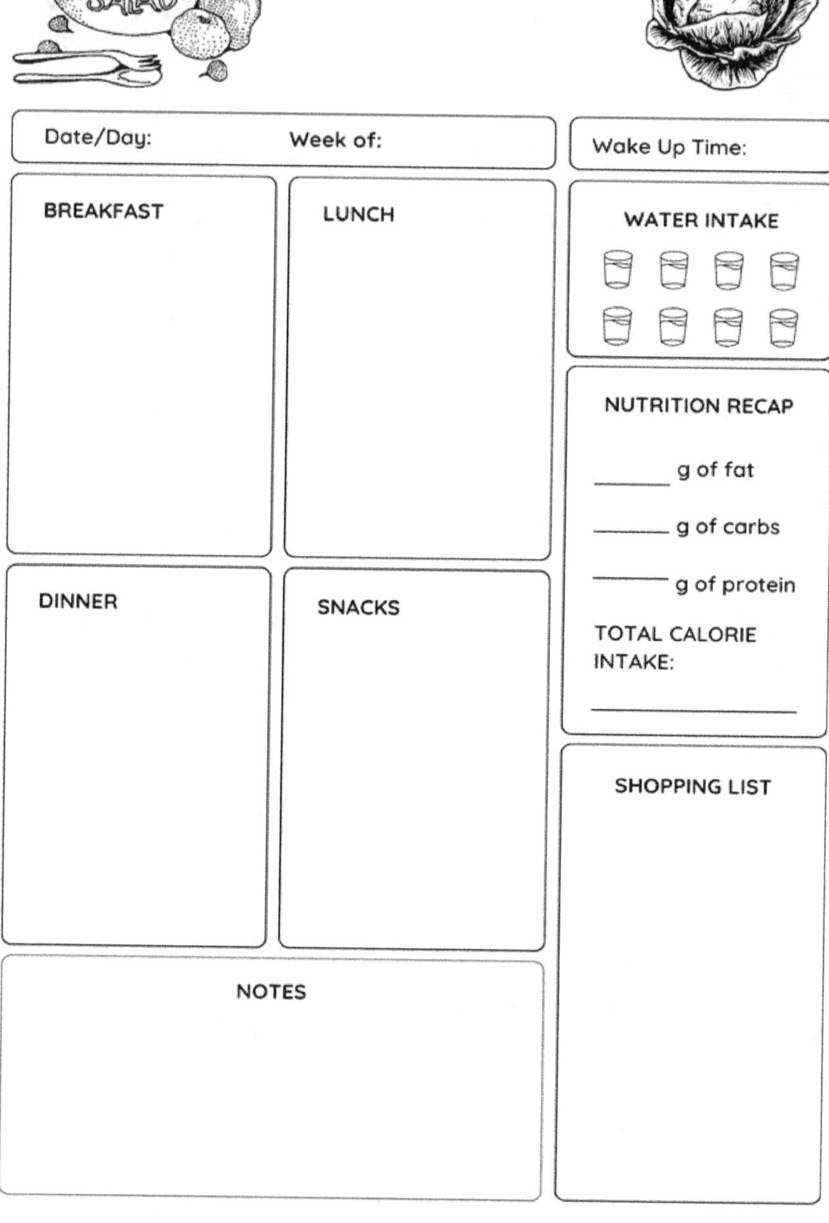

Date/Day: Week of:

Wake Up Time:

BREAKFAST

LUNCH

WATER INTAKE

NUTRITION RECAP

_________ g of fat

_________ g of carbs

_________ g of protein

TOTAL CALORIE INTAKE:

____

DINNER

SNACKS

SHOPPING LIST

NOTES